THE HOMEOPATH IN YOUR HAND

77 REMEDIES & HOW TO SELECT USING THEM
HOMEOPATHY HEALS™

By Lisa Strbac
LCHE BSc(Hons)

www.lisastrbac.com

For
J
R
G

&

Daisy

An introduction to this book

Hello,

Learning how to use homeopathy in the home is one of the most transformational steps an individual can make towards improving their health.

I have run successful workshops and courses to thousands of people and have been consistently asked by attendees to create a book based on my course including the top remedies to have at home. Whilst there are thousands of homeopathic remedies, this book covers what are, in my opinion, the most essential remedies to have in the home. I have also included my indispensable 'combination' remedies to have on hand in case you get stuck or are unsure what to give.

In total, this book guides you through 77 single/combination remedies and the foundations of homeopathy including how to select a remedy using my Homeopathy HEALS™ acronym. I created this to help people find remedies more easily and feedback was so great I wanted to include it in this book.

Homeopathy created a healthier life for me and my family - one where we are empowered and understand how to self treat common acute health issues. I truly believe that if everyone had a homeopathy kit and knew how to use it, society's mental and physical health would be transformed.

Lisa Strbac

Homeopath LCHE BSc(Hons) & Integrative Health Coach

> "
>
> 'The highest form of homeopathy is first aid prescribing. Almost every chronic case, if you take it back, where did it start? It started as a shock, with a grief, an accident, a medical procedure that went wrong. It started as a first aid situation and if that had been properly treated in the moment, someone had a home remedy kit and they knew what to do, this whole chain of health problems would never have needed to happen.'
> Ian Watson on Episode 35 of Raw Health Rebel Podcast with Lisa Strbac
>
> "

What is health?

Health is so much more than the absence of sickness. It is an inner contentment and sense of well-being. It is the ability to deal with stress and adapt to our environment.

When we are unable to maintain balance, for whatever reason (e.g. toxic overload, too much stress etc), our body produces symptoms as its way of communicating to us. We must always remember the innate wisdom of our body - symptoms are signals from the body and its way of trying to restore balance. Our symptoms often have a useful function, for example, a fever is its way of fighting off infection.

We all have this innate healing power which in homeopathy we call the 'Vital Force.' Homeopathy, via the use of remedies, provides the Vital Force with a message to stimulate self healing and restore homeostasis.

Homeopathy does not suppress symptoms which is why after using homeopathic remedies our bodies get stronger. When we suppress symptoms with allopathic medicines we can sometimes drive disease deeper. For example, there is a known link between steroid use for skin issues and the risk of later developing asthma. From a homeopathic perspective this is explained by the steroids simply suppressing symptoms. While they may remove the skin issues, they have not addressed the root cause. This suppression of symptoms drives the disease deeper with the body then producing more chronic lung symptoms, i.e. asthma.

Homeopathy works with the body's natural intelligence and only ever stimulates self healing.

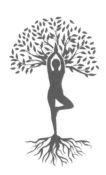

Why we do we get symptoms?

In order to understand why we get 'sick' it is useful to approach this depending on the nature of our symptoms.

Emergency/First Aid situations

Emergency and first aid situations occur due to very strong and intense exciting factors, which no matter how robust the individual's terrain is, can overwhelm a person's defences and set up their own state. In highly intense circumstances, such as a first aid trauma or accident, individuals are likely to react in a similar way. For example, if we cut ourselves; we will bleed, if we are accidentally hit with a hammer; we will bruise etc.

Acute illnesses

Acute illnesses are short term, self limiting illnesses such as colds, flu, vomiting, ear infection, throat infection, chicken pox, etc. They are a healthy response to an external stressor (which may be mental, emotional or physical). The stronger the stressor, the more similar the symptoms. We often get symptoms of sickness when we need to detox, whether that be emotionally or physically.

Individuality and susceptibility play a part in how we manifest our symptoms. For example, some people may be more prone to ear infections, while others may be more prone to respiratory complaints. The important thing to note is that when the body is supported through this dis-ease process, and symptoms are not suppressed, the body gets stronger.

Chronic illnesses

Chronic illnesses are long term health issues such as autoimmune problems, neurological issues and chronic infections etc. These are issues that are unable to resolve on their own due to a deep imbalance of the vital force. Disease starts from disturbances in the vital energy which then appear as physical symptoms. There are complex reasons as to why this happens, but it is often due to memories of past situations such as shock or trauma which can either be acquired in our own lifetime or even inherited. Always work with a homeopath when dealing with long term issues, as these need careful handling to peel back the contributing layers.

Introduction to Homeopathy

Homeopathy, the future of medicine, was discovered over 200 years ago by Dr Samuel Hahnemann (1755-1843). In a moment of inspired genius, Hahnemann made a connection between a natural plant medicine, cinchona bark, and the symptoms it produces. He realised that if a healthy individual takes cinchona bark, it produces symptoms of intermittent fever and malaria and yet if an individual who was sick with those same symptoms took cinchona bark it cured them. Homeopathy is founded on this 'like cures like' principle. A substance that can make a healthy person sick, can also make a sick person healthy.

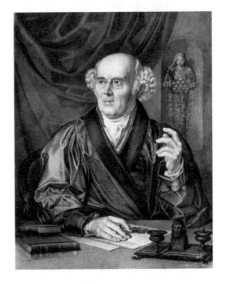

Dr. Samuel Hahnemann
1755 – 1843

Hahnemann found a way to 'potentise' the remedies so the toxic side effects of the medicinal substances were removed and yet they still worked just as, if not more, effectively.

The history of homeopathy is fascinating (and could warrant an entire book) - there is even a monument of Hahnemann in Washington, D.C.. This bronze statue of Hahnemann, sculpted by Charles Henry Niehaus, stands on a granite pedestal at Scott Circle. It was unveiled on 21 June 1900 and serves as a reminder of his contributions to medicine and the development of homeopathy.

The Flexner Report, published in 1910, had a profound impact on homeopathy particularly in the United States. It discredited homeopathy, leading to the closure of many homeopathic medical schools. As a result, homeopathy's use in mainstream medicine declined significantly. However, despite the report's criticism, homeopathy survived as an alternative medicine and continued to be used by many notable people including the UK's Royal Family (and just think for a moment how their wealth enables them to choose anything!). Today in the UK, King Charles III remains the Royal Patron of the Faculty of Homeopathy.

Homeopathy - Like cures like

Like cures like

The word homeopathy derives from the Greek words, 'homeo' meaning similar and 'pathos' meaning suffering, i.e. 'similar suffering.' Homeopathy is founded on the 'like cures like' principle, i.e. anything capable of producing symptoms of disease in a healthy person can cure those symptoms in a sick person.

To illustrate this principle of 'like cures like' consider what happens if a bee stings you. The affected area will sting and there may be a red, shiny painful lump. The homeopathic remedy made from the honeybee (Apis) is the number 1 remedy for bee stings and other bites or allergic reactions which produce a swollen, red and painful reaction.

In homeopathy we are always trying to find a remedy that best matches the individual's symptoms. In highly intense situations such as first aid trauma or shock, individuals will often react in a similar way and thus need similar homeopathic remedies.

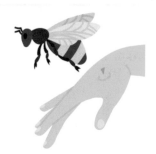

Example - Arsenicum

Arsenic (in its crude form)

The poison, if ingested in **material doses** causes the following toxic symptoms:

- vomiting
- diarrhea
- weakness
- chills
- collapse

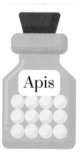

33   74.922

As

Arsenic

Arsenic in homeopathic form (called Arsenicum)

The poison, in **ultra-diluted homeopathic potency**, cures the same symptoms:

- vomiting
- diarrhea
- weakness
- chills
- collapse

How remedies are made

How are remedies made, i.e. 'potentised'?

Homeopathy is a form of energy medicine and homeopathic remedies are made by 'potentising' and 'succussing' the original substance - as illustrated below. This method removes any side effects from the original substance which could be of animal, plant or mineral origin. The succussing process (which means shaking) releases the energy of the substance.

One part of the original substance is mixed with 99 parts of liquid. This dilution is then succussed (i.e. shaken) to release the energy of the original substance to create a 1c potency (c stands for centesimal scale). Then 1 part of the 1c solution is diluted with another 99 parts of liquid and succussed again to create a 2c potency. This process is repeated until the desired potency is obtained. Most standard remedies come in 30c potency which means it has been through this dilution and succussion process 30 times.

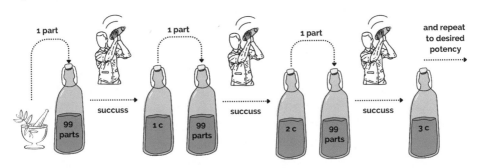

Although remedies are made in liquid they usually come in sugar pills which act as a carrier for the potentised remedy. A few drops of the homeopathic potentised liquid is added to the pills by the homeopathic manufacturer.

The laws of chemistry state that there is a limit to any dilution that can be made without losing the original substance altogether. This limit, which is related to Avogadro's number (6.023×1023), corresponds to homeopathic potencies of 12C. This is one of the reasons that mainstream science tries to discredit homeopathy, i.e. because there is no chemical substance left in potencies higher than 12c - **but homeopathy is based on physics NOT chemistry.**

Homeopathy is energy medicine

Remedies can be made from:

- Plants
- Minerals
- Animal derived
- Body derived ('sarcodes')
- Diseases ('nosodes')
- Imponderables (energy sources such as X-ray, sunlight, moonlight etc)

Remember how they are made - there is no material substance left. Homeopathy is based on energy not chemistry.

'Asking what is in the remedy is like asking what is 'in' a song....There is 'nothing' and yet there is everything in it.'

Lisa Strbac

Science is only just beginning to catch up with the possibilities of water carrying memory. In 2009, the Scientific Nobel prize winner, Dr. Luc Montagnier, and his team published a study in the journal 'Water,' where they reported detecting electromagnetic signals from highly diluted bacterial and viral DNA in water. They claimed that these signals could be transmitted to other water samples, even after the original DNA was no longer present due to extreme dilution. The researchers suggested that this phenomenon might explain the 'memory' of water and raised questions about the possible application of these findings to homeopathy.

'What I can say now is that the high dilutions are right. High dilutions of something are not nothing. They are water structures which mimic the original molecules.'

Dr Luc Montagnier

Potency

What potency?

- 30c is useful for most acute situations.
- 200c can be useful in extremely intense high energy situations such as emergencies and childbirth.
- Lower potencies such as 6 or 12c may need repeating more frequently than high potencies.
- If you have the 'right' remedy, regardless of what potency it is, it should trigger a self healing response.
- If it is the 'wrong' remedy then, regardless of potency, it will not trigger a healing response.
- 30c is a brilliant universal potency (which is why most homeopathy kits come with all remedies in a 30c). It crosses the bridge between mental and physical symptoms.

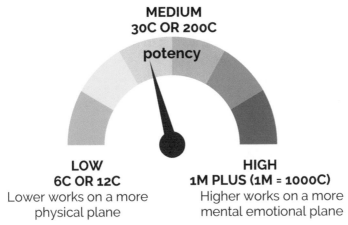

MEDIUM
30C OR 200C

potency

LOW
6C OR 12C
Lower works on a more
physical plane

HIGH
1M PLUS (1M = 1000C)
Higher works on a more
mental emotional plane

**In homeopathy the more the diluted, the more
energetic and thus more potent.**

Potency
<u>6 or 12c</u>
Stimulates physical healing.
<u>30c</u>
Heals on a physical and mental level.
<u>200c</u>
Sends a sharp, loud message. Useful in emergency acutes and used for constitutional prescribing.
<u>1m plus (1m = 1000c)</u>
Returns you back to self. Sends a deep but gentle message as to who you are. Used by professional homeopaths in constitutional prescribing.

**If in
doubt
use 30c**

How to choose a remedy

Individuality of symptoms

The remedy must fit the symptoms of the individual on an individual basis. Two people may have the same named condition, for example, the 'flu', but their experience of it and their symptoms might be very different. One person may have 'flu' with burning pains, restlessness and vomiting, the other person may feel dizzy, lethargic and tired. These two people will need different remedies to match their symptoms despite having the same allopathic label of 'flu.'

Homeopaths treat the individual, not the disease label.

To illustrate using a music analogy, think about how each individual responds differently to music. If you get the 'right' song in that moment, it could resonate to make an individual's hair stand on end. Yet the same song may not do anything for another person because it does not resonate. In homeopathy, we are always trying to find the remedy that resonates most with the individual.

How do I choose a remedy?

Each homeopathic remedy has its own individual essence, covering different mental and physical symptoms. The energy of the original substance is imprinted into the pills in a very special way due to the potentisation process. When the right remedy is found, energy can shift rapidly stimulating self healing.

The important concept in homeopathy is to find the right remedy to match the combination of symptoms the individual has. We can use homeopathy to self treat acute health issues using the '**Homeopathy HEALS**™' acronym to choose a remedy (see following page). Always work with a homeopath for help with chronic health issues as these can need careful handling to peel back the various contributing layers.

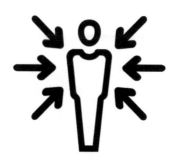

How to choose a remedy using Homeopathy HEALS ™

FOUR STEPS TO SELECT YOUR REMEDY

1. Extract 3-5 symptoms that are most specific and unusual using the **Homeopathy HEALS ™ technique** below.
2. Find your health issue in the symptoms index at the end of this book - if it is not listed choose the most similar issue.
3. Look up each remedy noted under the index and cross check the extracted 3-5 symptoms to the description of the remedies in this book.
4. Choose the remedy which best matches your symptoms. As long as the remedy matches your symptoms, it does not matter if you do not fit everything else the remedy may cover.

> The acronym HEALS was created by Lisa to help with remedy selection

Homeopathy HEALS ™

H is for Helps or Hinders - What helps the person feel better and what hinders healing? We can observe what is going on here. e.g. does the person feel better for lying down? or for fresh air? or company? or warmth/cold? etc or is the healing hindered by moving about? or warmth/cold? etc.

E is for Event – What event caused the complaint? Certain remedies have an affinity to certain events (or shocks). e.g. did it come on after being out in a cold dry wind (Aconite)? or after an accident (Arnica)? or after getting feet wet (Pulsatilla)?

A for Accompanying symptoms– What else is occurring alongside the main complaint? e.g. irritable, snotty nose, fever, thirstlessness

L is for Location - Be specific, find out where in the body the complaint is. Where exactly is it and where did it start? Is it the left side? the right side? or does it change?

S is for Sensations – What exactly does it feel like? e.g. needle, throbbing pain, pain worse for first movement.

Single homeopathic remedies can treat numerous ailments so it is highly unlikely you will cover every aspect of the remedy. As long as it is the best match for your 3-5 symptoms that is fine!

Example using Homeopathy HEALS™

Case example - 9 year old girl - ear infection of both ears - sometimes this one hurts more, sometimes the other, sometimes both. The girl is very weepy. She stops crying when spoken to - thus attentions helps. She had been splashing around in a puddle and 20 minutes later she came down with the ear infection. Nothing makes it worse. She is thirstless.

Step 1 - extract 3 - 5 symptoms for the ear infection using Homeopathy HEALS™ technique

    Helped or hindered by
    Helped by attention
    Event that caused
    Getting feet wet
    Accompanying symptoms
    Thirstless
    Weeping
    Location
    Changing sides
    Sensation
    Nothing notable

Step 2 - Look up the health issue in the index - if it is not listed choose the most similar issue.

Step 3 - Look up each remedy noted under the index and cross check the extracted 3-5 symptoms to the remedies in this book - see example below.

Remedies listed under ear infection	SYMPTOMS					
	Helped by attention	Getting feet wet	Thirst-less	Weeping	Changeable symptoms	Total score
Aconite	0	0	0	0	0	0
Belladonna	0	0	1	0	0	1
Calc Carb	0	0	0	0	0	0
Chamomilla	0	0	0	0	0	0
Ferrum Phos	0	0	0	0	0	0
Hepar Sulph	0	0	0	0	0	0
Merc	0	0	0	0	0	0
Pulsatilla	1	1	1	1	1	5
Silica	0	0	0	0	0	0

Step 4 - Choose the remedy which best matches 3-5 symptoms by looking up the remedy description in this book. The best matched remedy in the above example is **Pulsatilla.**

Template for Homeopathy HEALS™

Step 1 - extract 3 - 5 symptoms for the health issue using Homeopathy HEALS™ technique.

Step 2 - Look up the health issue in the index - if it is not listed choose the most similar issue.

Step 3 - Look up each remedy noted under the index and cross check the extracted 3-5 symptoms to the remedies in this book.

Helped or hindered by

_____

_____

Event that caused

_____

Accompanying symptoms

_____

_____

Location

_____

Sensation

_____

	SYMPTOMS						
Remedies listed in index for issue							Total score

Step 4 - Choose the remedy which best matches your symptoms. As long as the remedy matches your symptoms it does not matter if you do not fit everything else the remedy may cover. **Single homeopathic remedies treat numerous ailments so you will not match every aspect of the remedy.**

How to choose a remedy
Homeopathy HEALS™prompts

H Helped or Hindered by

- BODY FUNCTION - sleeping, eating, drinking, sweating, urinating, bowel motion, coughing, sneezing, sex, yawning, sleep.
- ENVIRONMENT - sun, fog, damp, storms, weather. changes, clear, outside, inside, windows open, breeze.
- MOVEMENT - first movement, any movement, continued movement, gentle motion, stretching, bending forward/backward, pressure, rest, exertion.
- POSITION - lying down, on the side, one side, sitting up, being carried, stooping.
- PSYCHOLOGICAL- excitement, being busy, studying, company, being alone.
- SENSES - sound, music, touch, lights, pressure, smells.
- TEMPERATURE - heat, cold, change of temperature, hot compress, cold bathing,
- TIME - specific time of day, day vs night, full moon, seasons, weekly, monthly, during menses.

Helped by is denoted by > (makes better or ameliorated by)
Hindered by is denoted by < (worse for or aggravated by)

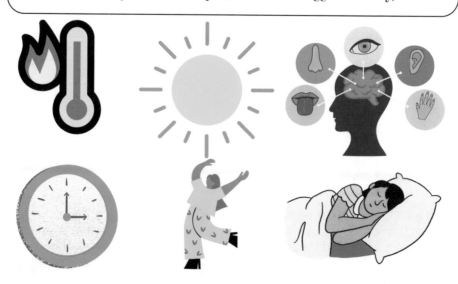

How to choose a remedy
Homeopathy HEALS™ prompts

E Event that caused symptoms

- Abandonment?
- Abuse?
- Accident?
- Alcohol?
- Anger?
- Bad news?
- Childbirth?
- Drugs?
- Fall?
- Food poisoning?
- Grief?
- Head injury?
- Heartache?
- Homesickness?
- Hormonal changes?
- Jealousy?
- Medication?
- Never been well since an illness?
- Over studying?
- Shock?
- Stress?
- Teething?
- Weather - getting wet, chilled, draft, wind, summer?

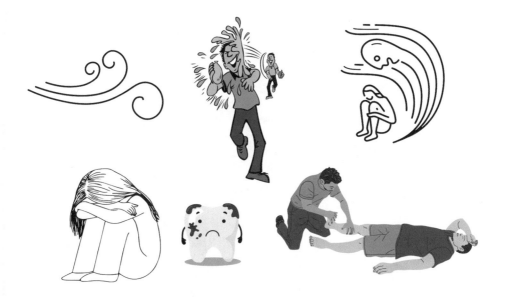

How to choose a remedy
Homeopathy HEALS™prompts

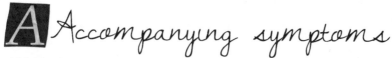

A Accompanying symptoms

What other symptoms are there as well as the main complaint?

Examples such as:

- Sweating?
- Shivering?
- Hot face?
- Cold or hot feet/hands?
- Discharges?
- Taste in the mouth?
- Thirsty?
- Irritable?
- Clingy?
- Weeping?
- Wants to be left alone?
- Lethargy?
- Appetite?

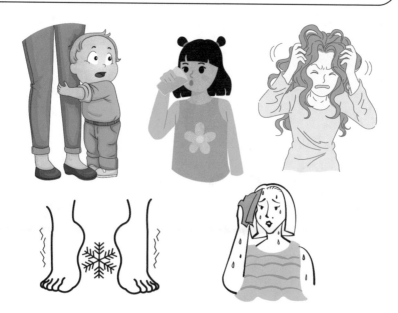

How to choose a remedy
Homeopathy HEALS™ prompts

L *Location*

- Where in the body is the complaint?
- Right sided?
- Left sided?
- Did it move from one side to the other?
- Did it start in one place and move somewhere else?
- Does it change?
- Does it radiate?
- Head - top, side, middle, bottom?
- Ears - just ears or ears and throat?
- Throat - right side of throat, middle or left?
- Be as specific as possible

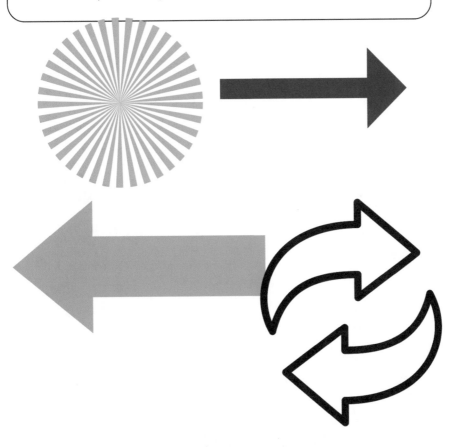

S Sensations

- Throbbing or pulsating
- Bone breaking
- Stiffness, constricted or numbness
- Sharp - cutting, stabbing, stitching, pricking, splinter like, stinging
- Darting, shooting, lancinating, digging, drawing, pulling
- Aching, dull, sore, bruised
- Crushing
- Spasmodic, cramping or jerking
- Boring, twisting, pinching, gnawing, tearing
- Nauseating
- Weakness
- Burning, heat or coldness of part
- Bubbling or boiling
- As if something loose, expanded or separate from the body
- Trembling or twitching
- Erratic, consistent, spreading or changeable pain

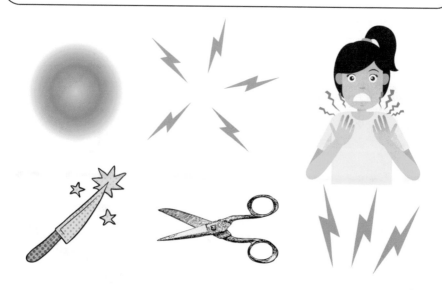

What does healing look like?

Healing does not always look like an instant disappearance of symptoms. Some symptoms have a function, such as a fever, and while homeopathy will speed up the innate healing process, it will not instantly remove symptoms which are useful.

The Law of Cure (Hering's Law of Cure)
The Law of Cure is named after Constantine Hering who was a prominent homeopathic physician (1800-1880). He observed clear patterns of healing that can take place during homeopathic treatment as noted below.

Hering's Law of Cure

TOP TO BOTTOM
Symptoms may move from top to bottom, or from the centre to extremities. E.g. joint pains or rashes may move from shoulders to hips, then to legs.

FROM INSIDE TO OUTSIDE
Symptoms move from within to out. We must allow the body to cleanse and eliminate toxins without suppressing any kind of discharge.

REVERSE ORDER
Old symptoms which have been suppressed or incompletely cured may return, and in the reverse order of their original appearance.

FROM MOST IMPORTANT TO LEAST IMPORTANT ORGANS
E.g. as depression/anxiety/panic attacks clears the patient may develop symptoms on a physical level such as a rash or digestive disorders.

You feel better - pain and symptoms subside. You have more energy.

You may fall asleep - the body gets to work while you sleep and you wake up feeling better.

Elimination may occur - discharges such as mucus, diarrhoea, vomit, rashes, profuse urination or even words occur temporarily and you feel better after.

 Please be sensible and use your judgement. If healing is not happening or there are red flags, always seek urgent medical advice.

How to dose remedies

THE LAW OF THE MINIMUM DOSE - Less is more!
Generally, give one pill and WAIT to see results and assess the effects of the remedy. If you feel much better after a dose, stop taking the remedy until the first sign that your symptoms have returned. You can keep repeating the remedy until a definite improvement is maintained.

When do I repeat the remedy?
Repeat the remedy when improvement stalls or the same symptoms return. In intense acute situations you may need to repeat the remedy frequently because the 'energy' of the remedy may be used up by the body more quickly.

What if nothing has happened?
If you have taken 3-4 doses and there is no improvement it may be a sign that a different remedy is needed. It is fine to try a new remedy if the first one did not help at all.

What if my symptoms change?
If symptoms change then it is ok to change remedies (but remember some remedies, such as Pulsatilla, do have changeable symptoms as part of their picture).

When will I feel better?
The pace of the illness determines how quickly you can expect the remedies to work - for example, an individual with a migraine should respond quickly, whereas something like slow onset flu symptoms or chicken pox will take more time.

ALWAYS STOP TAKING REMEDIES ONCE YOU FEEL BETTER

The Homeopathic Law of the 'Minimum Dose' says you should take the smallest number of doses. The remedy only initiates self healing, so once that process has commenced, you can let the body do the rest. Always remember the innate wisdom of your body and what an incredible self healing machine it is.

 Please be sensible and use your judgement. If healing is not happening or it is a medical emergency, please seek help from an appropriate healthcare professional.

Dosing guidelines for acute illnesses

> Dosing homeopathic remedies can take some getting used to because, unlike with allopathic Western medicine, there are no set regimes or protocols. It is crucial to listen to the body and to see how it responds to the remedy. Depending on the individual and the nature of the symptoms, sometimes just one dose is all that is needed, yet at other times the remedy may need repeating frequently such as every 15 minutes. Below are some general dosing guidelines for intense acute illnesses.

DOSING GUIDELINES:

- Remember to ALWAYS LISTEN TO THE BODY
- Give every 15-60 minutes and reduce as the symptoms improve
- STOP when definite improvement is maintained
- If you have given 3-4 doses and there is NO improvement then try a different remedy
- If symptoms do return, resume giving the remedy

POTENCY:

- Ideally use 30c - it is a brilliant universal potency
- 12c can be used if 30c is not available but it may need repeating more often
- 200c can be suitable for high intensity acute situations especially where there are strong mental symptoms, such as childbirth

 ALWAYS STOP TAKING THE REMEDIES ONCE YOU FEEL BETTER

Frequently asked questions

Can I take more than one remedy at the same time?

Ideally just use one remedy at a time so that you can properly assess the reaction of the remedy. However, use your judgement - for example, in an emergency it would be fine to use Arnica and Aconite alternating in quick succession. There are some amazing combination remedies which work in beautiful harmony together. This book covers the top ones to have at home.

What potency?

30c is useful for most acute situations. 200c can be useful in extremely intense high energy situations, such as emergencies and childbirth. Lower potencies such as 6 or 12c may need repeating more frequently than high potencies. 30c is a brilliant universal potency. The remedy is much more important than the potency.

How many pills should I take?

Remember, homeopathy is energy medicine and very different from Western allopathic medicine. In homeopathy, it is the FREQUENCY of administering that counts as a dose; the pill is just a vessel for the energy of the substance so it doesn't matter whether you give one, three or 10 pills when taken at the same time. Give just one pill to make the bottle/tube/packet of remedies last longer!

Is homeopathy safe and can it be used for babies or during pregnancy?

Yes, homeopathy is safe for newborns and during pregnancy and while breastfeeding. Remember these remedies only contain the energetic profile of the original substances. If you take the wrong remedy it simply will not work and as long as you do not continuously take it when not needed, it will do no harm.

How do I administer to a baby or someone who doesn't like the pills?

It is possible to 'water dose' remedies when administering to babies or those that don't like the pills. Simply dissolve one pill in water (or breast milk). The volume of water/milk that the remedy is dissolved in does not matter. One drop of that liquid then counts as one dose. You can keep the potentised liquid solution for 24-48 hours. This is a great way to also make a remedy last longer if you are down to your last pill and think you'll need multiple doses over a short period of time.

Frequently asked questions

Can I eat or drink after taking the remedies?
Ideally give 15 minutes away from food and drink and especially after cleaning teeth or drinking coffee.

How should I store my remedies?
Homeopathic remedies are energy medicine and should ideally be stored away from wifi. Keep away from strong smells and essential oils such as camphor, menthol and eucalyptus which can antidote the remedies.

Does it matter if I chew the remedy?
No, it does not matter. It will still work just fine if you chew the remedy.

Can I touch the remedies?
Remedies are delicate - touch as little as possible. Shake one pill into the lid and put straight into the mouth if possible. Alternatively, you can crush the remedy and put into water and sip - remember ONE SIP EQUALS ONE DOSE.

I felt so good on the remedy can I keep taking it?
Remember the Minimum Dose. Less is more with homeopathy! If you continually take a homeopathic remedy when it is not needed, you may experience a proving (highly unlikely in acute situations). Any symptoms produced during a proving resolve once the remedy is stopped.

What is a proving?
A proving is the homeopathic method of testing a substance on a healthy person. In a homeopathic proving, a homeopathic remedy is administered to healthy volunteers in order to produce the symptoms specific to that substance and thereby reveal its curative powers. If we continually take a homeopathic remedy when we are in a healthy state we risk proving the remedy. This is why we should only take homeopathic remedies when we have symptoms and only take the minimum dose. Even if remedies are proved, symptoms will stop as soon as you stop taking the remedy.

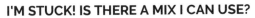

I'M STUCK! IS THERE A MIX I CAN USE?
Where relevant, each health issue noted in the index will have a 'mix', also known as a 'combination remedy', listed which can be used when you're unsure.

Essential single remedies

Aconite	Hepar Sulph
Aecsulus	Histaminum
Allium Cepa	Hypericum
Ambra Grisea	Ignatia
Anacardium	Ipecac
Ant Tart	Kali Bich
Apis	Kali Carb
Arg Nit	Kali Phos
Arnica	Lachesis
Arsenicum	Ledum
Belladonna	Lycopodium
Bellis Perennis	Mag Phos
Bryonia	Merc
Calc Carb	Mixed Pollens
Calc Phos	Nat Mur
Calendula	Nux Vomica
Candida Albicans	Opium
Cantharis	Phos Ac
Capsicum	Phosphorus
Carbo Veg	Phytolacca
Caulophyllum	Pulsatilla
Causticum	Rhus Tox
Chamomilla	Ruta
Chelidonium	Sabadilla
China	Secale
Cimicifiuga	Sepia
Cina	Silica
Cocculus	Spongia
Colocynthis	Staphisagria
Dolichos	Stramonium
Drosera	Streptococcinum
Eupatorium	Sulphur
Euphrasia	Thuja
Ferrum Phos	Tuberculinum
Gelsemium	

Aconite
Nipping colds in the bud, sudden inflammation, panic

KEY SYMPTOMS:
- Sudden, violent onset
- 1st stage inflammation
- Palpitations
- Panic attacks
- Very sensitive to noise, touch or smell
- High fever
- Unbearable pain (can scream)
- Unquenchable thirst - everything tastes bitter except water

acute, sudden, violent onset

burning thirst for cold drinks

sensitive to noise & smell

intolerable pain

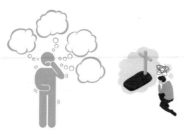

restless & anxious - may fear death

MENTAL SYMPTOMS
Very anxious
Fearful
May fear death
May say 'I want to die' with pain

EVENT THAT CAUSED SYMPTOMS:
Fright or shock
Sudden and violent changes in weather
Chilled by dry, cold weather or draft

ailments after cold wind

shock

< midnight

> rest

Hindered by:
Touch
Light
Noise
Being chilled by cold wind
Dry weather
12am-2am
Warm room

Helped by:
Open air
Warm sweat
Rest
Sleep

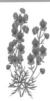

HELP!

Aconite
Cheat sheet

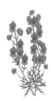

Full name: Aconitum Napellus
Other names: Monkshood, Wolfsbane
Found growing in damp Mountainous areas in Europe, Central Asia and Europe. It is a distinctive looking wildflower on shoulder high sturdy stems.

USEFUL FOR:

ACUTE ANXIETY: Panic attacks, sudden onset fear and trembling. Fear of death and extreme terror. Use as a tranquilizer before or after a fearful event. Palpitations.

COUGH: Hoarse, dry, painful cough or short barking cough. Hindered by inhaling. Worse at night.

CROUP: Use in early stages, normally starts around midnight. If fails to help then alternate Hepar Sulph and Spongia.

EARLY STAGE INFECTIONS: Use at first sign of a cold, flu, sore throat or ear infection. May have come on after a shock or being in a cold dry wind.

EAR: Earache with pain. May be tingling and buzzing or feel like a drop of water is in the ear. Sensitive to noises, music is unbearable.

FEVERS: Cold feet and hot hands. Tremendous thirst. One or both cheeks flushed. Fever alternates with chills. Pupils constricted. Restlessness and anxiety.

FLU: Sudden, violent onset. Thirsty.

HEART ATTACK (seek urgent medical advice, take remedy while waiting for help): with chest pain, radiating pain, numbness in left arm. Fear of death (also take Arnica)

TRAUMA AND ITS AFTER EFFECTS (also take Arnica): Helps with emotional shock.

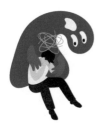

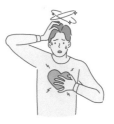

Aesculus
Backache, hemorrhoids, hip joint pain, varicose veins

KEY SYMPTOMS:

- Hemorrhoids with much pain but little bleeding
- Everything slowed down - from digestion to heart
- Sensation of fullness in parts
- Any pain or aching in pelvis or hips
- Degenerative hip disease
- Sensation of heat, dryness, stiffness and roughness
- Walking greatly aggravates
- Backache worse for stooping
- Spine feels weak
- Throbbing behind pubis
- Lameness of back
- Burning in anus - feels full of small sticks

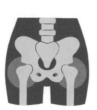

pain in pelvis or hips

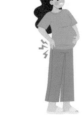

backache

hemorrhoids

sensation of heat

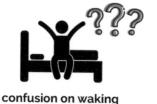

confusion on waking

MENTAL SYMPTOMS
Depressed
Irritable
Wakes up with confusion

EVENT THAT CAUSED SYMPTOMS:
None to note

< walking

> bathing

Hindered by:
Walking
Stooping
On waking
After stool

Helped by:
Bleeding
In Summer
Bathing

Aesculus
Cheat sheet

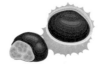

Full name: Aesculus Hippocastanum
Other names: Horse chestnut
The horse chestnut is native to South East Europe but it has been widely cultivated across the world. It can now be found in Europe, North America and other temperate regions worldwide.

USEFUL FOR:

BACK PAIN: Hindered by walking and stooping. Spine feels weak. Worse in sacrum and hip area. Back which gives out in pregnancy. Herniated and ruptured discs.

CONSTIPATION: Large, hard stools, followed by feeling of prolapse.

FEMALE: Throbbing behind pubis.

HEMORRHOIDS: Burning in anus. Dryness - feels full of small sticks or as if a bug crawling in the anus. Hemorrhoids with much pain but little bleeding. Chills up and down the back. Pain after stool with prolapse. Sharp shooting pains up the back. Worse during menopause. Hemorrhoids like a bunch of grapes. Relieved by bleeding.

JOINT PAINS: Degenerative hip disease. Aching. Bruised sensation. Feels as if legs may give way. Pain shooting down arms. Numb fingertips. Worse in the morning on waking and for movement.

LIVER: Soreness and fullness in the liver region.

VARICOSE VEINS: may be purple in colour. Fullness. Dry, swollen mucus membranes.

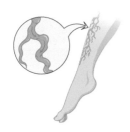

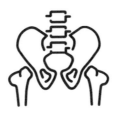

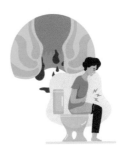

Allium Cepa
Colds, hayfever

KEY SYMPTOMS:
- Colds
- Hayfever
- Acrid nasal discharges
- Bland tears
- Burning of the eyelids, nose, mouth, throat, bladder and skin
- Burning eyelids
- Hacking cough on inhaling cold air
- Oppressed breathing
- Watery discharge with sneezing

burning

burning of eyelids

acrid nasal discharges

oppressed breathing

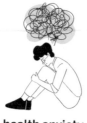

health anxiety

MENTAL SYMPTOMS
Health anxiety
Despair of recovery

EVENT THAT CAUSED SYMPTOMS:
Damp cold wind
Wet feet
Spring (colds)
August (hayfever)

cold wind

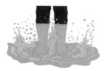

wet feet

< warm room

> cold room

Hindered by:
Warm room
Damp
Spring
Wet feet
Singing

Helped by:
Open air
Cold room
Bathing
Motion

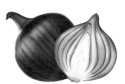

HELP! Allium Cepa
Cheat sheet

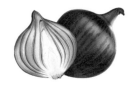

Other names: Red onion, Alliaceae
Red onions are cultivated in various parts of the world, including Europe, North America, Asia and the Mediterranean region. They have been traditionally used in medicine for their potential anti-inflammatory, antimicrobial, cardiovascular, respiratory and digestive health benefits.

USEFUL FOR:

ALLERGIES: Nose drips. Watery nasal discharge which may burn. Sneezing. Watery bland tears. Itching in the back of the throat. Hindered by warm rooms. Helped by fresh air. Allergies every August.

COLDS: Sneezing. Acrid burning discharges from nose. Watery profuse discharges which burn the nose and upper lip. Coughs which are worse in a warm room and helped by open air. Spring colds.

HAYFEVER: Bland watery eyes, acrid nasal discharge (opposite from Euphrasia). Nose drips. Watery nasal discharge which may burn. Sneezing. Watery bland tears. Hindered by warm rooms. Helped by fresh air. Hayfever every August. Burning of the eyelids and nose.

NERVE PAIN: Neuralgic pains like a fine thread. May occur following an amputation or injury to nerves, Left sided facial paralysis. Symptoms go from left to right,

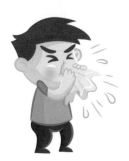

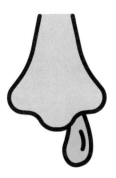

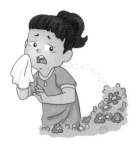

Ambra Grisea
Anxiety, coughs, potty training problems

KEY SYMPTOMS:

- Extreme nervous hypertension
- Twitches and jerking
- Cannot urinate or pass stool in front of others
- Blushes easily
- Numbness in arms
- Spasmodic, barking cough
- Palpitations as if chest obstructed
- Insomnia due to worry
- Bloating of stomach
- Sensation of coldness in abdomen
- Impaired hearing
- Symptoms change place

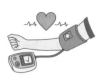

nervous hypertension

cannot urinate in front of others

palpitations

barking cough

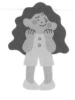

shy

MENTAL SYMPTOMS
Intensely shy
Time passes slowly
Slow comprehension

EVENT THAT CAUSED SYMPTOMS:
Business failure
Deaths in family
Shock

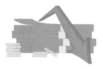

business failure

deaths

< presence of others

> cold drinks

Hindered by:
Music
Presence of others
Thinking of problems
Morning
Warmth

Helped by:
Slow motion
Open air
Cold drinks

HELP! Ambra Grisea
Cheat sheet

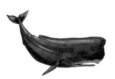
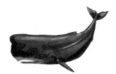

Other names: Ambergris, Morbid secretion of the whale
A substance formed in the digestive system of sperm whales in response to irritants. It is highly valued in the perfume industry for its unique fragrance and is collected from the ocean's surface after being expelled by the whales.

USEFUL FOR:

ANXIETY: Nervous hypertension - weakened by age or overwork. Extreme shyness. Cannot urinate or pass stool in front of others (potty training issues). Blushes easily. Loss of love for life. Music may cause weeping. Hindered by company.

BLADDER: Feels as if only a few drops or urine passes. Cannot pass urine in front of others.

COUGHS: Nervous barking or spasmodic cough. Tickling in throat.

HEADACHE: Tearing pain in upper half of brain. Brain feels loose. Rush of blood to head especially when listening to music.

INSOMNIA: Cannot sleep due to worry. Tired when goes to bed yet wakes as soon as head hits the pillow. Twitching of limbs during sleep.

PALPITATIONS: Palpitations in chest as if chest obstructed or a lump lodged.

TWITCHES AND JERKS: Nerves affected causing jerks and twitching. Weakness, coldness or numbness in fingers or arms. Trembling of lower part.

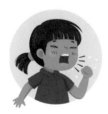
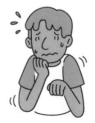
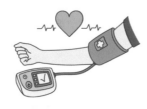

Anacardium
Exam nerves, nervous exhaustion, headaches

KEY SYMPTOMS:

- Exam nerves
- Nervous exhaustion from overstudy
- Poor memory
- Headaches hindered by mental exertion and helped by eating
- Antidote to poison oak and ivy
- Sensation of plug in various parts
- Emptiness in stomach
- Eating temporarily relieves issues
- Thirst during fever

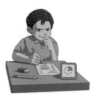

exam nerves

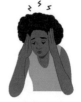

headaches

poison ivy

sensation of plug in various parts

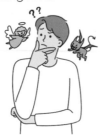

devil on one shoulder angel on the other

MENTAL SYMPTOMS

Feels as if a devil on one shoulder and angel on the other
Manic depression
May curse and swear
Easily offended

EVENT THAT CAUSED SYMPTOMS:

Verbal or physical abuse
Humiliation
Examinations

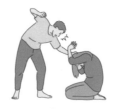

abuse

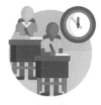

exams

< mental exertion

> eating

Hindered by:
Mental exertion
Hot water
Strong smells
Motion

Helped by:
Eating
Lying on side
Hot bath
Sunshine

Anacardium
Cheat sheet

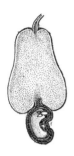

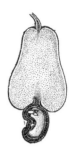

Full name: Anacardium Orientale
Other names: Marking nut, Malacca bean
The marking nut is native to India and is found in other parts of South East Asia as well. It is a small, kidney-shaped nut that contains a caustic oil called cardol, which can cause skin irritation and blistering.

USEFUL FOR:

ANXIETY: Fear of examinations. Lack of confidence. Fear of the future. Fear or impending misfortune. Hypochondria. Fear of being poisoned.

EXHAUSTION: Overwork and brain fatigue. Nervous exhaustion from overstudy. Absentminded and forgetful. Suddenly forgets thoughts,. Lack of mental and physical power.

HEADACHES: Headache from overstudy. Nervous headaches. Pressing pain, as if a plug, in forehead. Helped by eating.

STOMACH: Loss of appetite. Refuses to eat for fear of being poisoned. Empty feeling in stomach. Eating temporarily helps.

POISON IVY OR OAK RASH: Intense itching. Weals. Yellowish fluid.

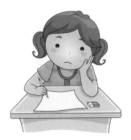

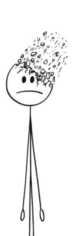

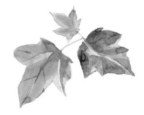

Ant Tart
Breathlessness, chest issues, flu

KEY SYMPTOMS:

- Rattling of chest
- Lots of mucus but can't cough it up
- Weak and drowsy
- Rattling, loose cough
- Breathless
- Pale face with cold sweat
- Quivering of lower jaw and chin
- Desires apples
- Thirsty for cold water, little and often
- Nausea with retching

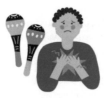

rattling sounds in chest

difficult fast breathing

chest full of mucus but can't cough it up

low vitality

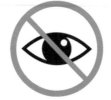

does not want to be looked at

MENTAL SYMPTOMS

Does not want to be looked at
Despondency
Fear of being alone

EVENT THAT CAUSED SYMPTOMS:

Anger
Damp

anger

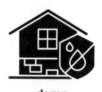

damp

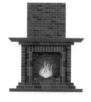

< warmth

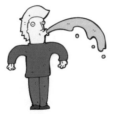

> expectoration

Hindered by:
Warmth (rooms, weather)
Anger
Lying down

Helped by:
Expectoration
Sitting erect
Vomiting

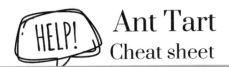

Ant Tart
Cheat sheet

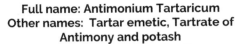

Full name: Antimonium Tartaricum
Other names: Tartar emetic, Tartrate of Antimony and potash
Made from the compound antimony potassium tartrate, also known as tartar emetic. It is a white, odourless powder that is derived from a reaction between antimony oxide and potassium bitartrate (cream of tartar).

USEFUL FOR:

COUGHS: Gasps for air before coughing attack. Loose rattling cough. Cough may be followed by vomiting.

NAUSEA: Nausea with difficulty vomiting. Sickness felt in the chest. Vomits thick white mucus which may be streaked with blood. Thirstless and may vomit water if they try to drink it.

RESPIRATORY: Rattling of mucus. Lungs seem full of mucus but unable to cough it up. Gasping for air. Shortness of breath. Nostrils flare. Severe pneumonia at the end stages. Thin white mucus.

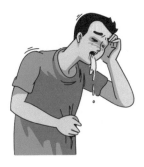

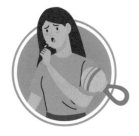

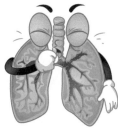

Apis
Stings, bites, hives, sore throats, cystitis

KEY SYMPTOMS:
- Burning
- Stinging
- Itching
- Swelling and puffiness
- Shiny and red
- Right sided complaints or right to left
- Flushes of heat
- Stinging sore throat
- Stinging at start of urination
- Frequent urge to urinate
- Thirstless

burning

puffiness & swelling

stinging & red

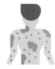

itching

active & busy

MENTAL SYMPTOMS
Active and busy
Restless
Weeping

EVENT THAT CAUSED SYMPTOMS:
Jealousy
Fright
Rage
Insect bite

jealousy

Insect bite

< heat

> cold applications

Hindered by:
Touch (even of hair)
Pressure
Heat
Lying down
4pm
Right eye

Helped by:
Cold applications
Motion
Fresh air
Sitting up

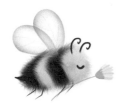

HELP!

Apis
Cheat sheet

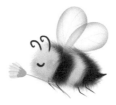

Full name: Apis Mellifica
Other names: Honeybee
Apis is prepared from the sting of the
common honeybee.

USEFUL FOR:
ALLERGIES: Swelling with stinging, burning, sharp pains and itching.
Redness and swelling.

BLADDER: Cystitis with scalding pain during urination. Nephritis with
swelling everywhere and scanty urine.

COLD SORES: Especially the left side helped by cold applications.

EYES: Styes. Conjunctivitis. May have swollen lids which can hardly
be forced open.

SKIN ISSUES: Hives, insect bites or urticaria with burning pains. Bright
red swelling, tense edema of skin. Redness, burning, shiny red.
Burns. Helped by cold applications

SHINGLES: Burning, stinging and itching

THROAT: Sore throat, Scarlet fever, tonsillitis. With redness, swelling,
helped by cold food or drinks. Throat pain extending to ears.

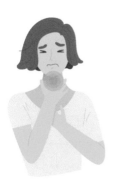

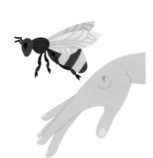

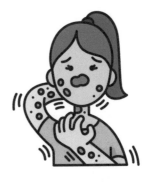

Arg Nit
Anticipatory anxiety, diarrhoea

KEY SYMPTOMS:
- Anticipatory anxiety, fear & panic
- Flatulence, gas and bloating
- Diarrhoea from anticipation
- Headache - feels like head is expanding
- Sore throat - splinter like pain
- Palpitations
- Conjunctivitis with discharge
- Coughs caused by high notes
- Vertigo looking down from heights
- Spinach coloured stools
- Craves fresh air and space
- Desires sugar but worse for it
- Hypoglycemia
- Coldness and trembling

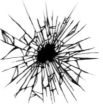

gas & bloating

nervous diarrhoea

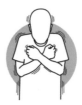

splinter like pains

coldness & trembling

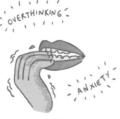

anxiety

MENTAL SYMPTOMS
Anxious and overthinking
Hurried
Performance anxiety

EVENT THAT CAUSED SYMPTOMS:
Anticipation
Mental strain
Sugar

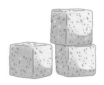

anticipation

sugar

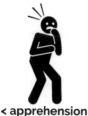
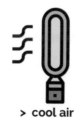

< apprehension

> cool air

Hindered by:
Apprehension
Warm rooms
Left side
Looking down

Helped by:
Cool air
Cold bath

Full name: Argentum Nitricum
Other names: Silver nitrate, Lunar caustic
The homeopathic remedy Arg Nit is made from the compound silver nitrate. Silver nitrate is a chemical compound that is a colourless, crystalline solid which is highly soluble in water.

USEFUL FOR:

ANXIETY: Anticipatory anxiety. Fear before dentist or doctor. Fear of flying or heights. Fears having a panic attack. Performance anxiety. Diarrhoea from thinking about upcoming events. Thinks that she will fail.

EYES: Conjunctivitis where eyelids may be stuck together. Lots of discharge. Photophobia. Thick crusts on eyelids.

HEADACHES: Nervous headache with trembling. Sensation of expanding. Coldness. Helped by tight bandaging and pressure.

SORE THROAT: Sensation as if splinter in the throat. Thick mucus in throat. Burning and dryness. Difficult swallowing. Chronic laryngitis of singers. High notes can cause cough.

STOMACH: Diarrhoea from emotions or anticipation. Loose stools from eating too much sugar or candy. Fluids seem to pass straight through. Flatulence, Colic with distension and gas. Rumbling tummy. Indigestion with belching and bloating.

VERTIGO: Vertigo at the sight of high buildings or looking down from heights.

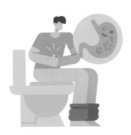
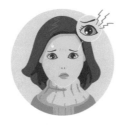
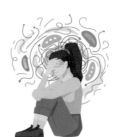

Arnica
Universal trauma remedy, accidents, shock, collapse

KEY SYMPTOMS:
- Injuries and pain
- Shock and trauma - mental or emotional
- Bleeding including gums
- Bruised, aching and soreness
- Crushing pains - bed feels hard
- Head injury-concussion
- Palpitations
- Post exertion
- Stroke, heart attacks and suspected clots
- Drowsiness
- Collapse
- Lack of oxygen

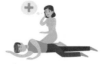

universal trauma remedy

bleeding

bruised feeling

pain

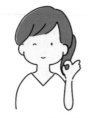

may say 'I'm fine'

MENTAL SYMPTOMS
May say 'I am fine': 'nothing wrong with me'
Underestimates the severity of the trauma.

EVENT THAT CAUSED SYMPTOMS:
Injury
Blood loss

injury

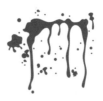

blood loss

< overexertion

> lying down

Hindered by:
Overexertion
Morning
Motion
Damp cold
Alcohol
After sleep

Helped by:
Lying down
Head low
Out stretched

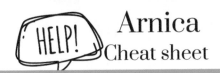 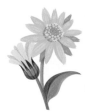

Arnica
Cheat sheet

HELP!

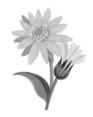

Full name: Arnica Montana
Other names: Leopard's bane, mountain daisy, mountain tobacco
Arnica is probably the most well known homeopathic remedy. Found growing in the mountains of Central Europe. This plant grows naturally where accidents and injuries can occur, illustrating how 'nature provides.'

First choice in any emergency or first aid situation

USEFUL FOR:

ANY TRAUMA OR ACCIDENT: First choice after most accidents, physical ordeals or injuries. Provides pain relief. Helps with bruising. Use for head injuries, concussion and any sprains, strains or overexertion.

JET LAG: Can help mild trauma caused by disorientation in jet lag.

JOINT PAINS: Sore and bruised sensation. May be sensitive to touch.

HEART ATTACKS, COLLAPSE, SUSPECTED BLOOD CLOTS AND STROKE: seek urgent medical advice, take remedy while waiting for help.

POST SURGERY, POST LABOUR AND DENTAL PROCEDURES: To help speed up healing.

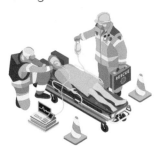

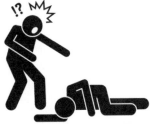

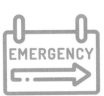

Arsenicum
Food poisoning, flu, anxiety

KEY SYMPTOMS:
- Cold, chilly and craves heat
- Fastidiousness
- Burning pains relieved by heat
- Diarrhoea, stomach pain
- Vomiting
- Hayfever with burning discharges
- Thirsty for small frequent sips
- Extreme weakness yet restless
- Offensive discharges
- Discharges watery, smelly, burning
- Likes hot drinks and food

weakness &
extreme
fatigue

burning pains
relieved by heat

chilly

burning discharges

anxiety
desires company

MENTAL SYMPTOMS
Anxiety desires company
Worried about health
May have fear of death
Despair of recovery

EVENT THAT CAUSED SYMPTOMS:
Food poisoning
Loss of finances
Getting chilled

food poisoning

loss of finances

< midnight

> warmth

Hindered by:
Ice
Cold food
Cold air
After midnight
Tobacco
Lying on the affected part

Helped by:
Hot dry applications
Hot food/drinks
Warmth
Walking about
Company
Sitting upright
Elevating head

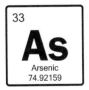

Arsenicum
Cheat sheet

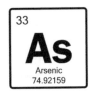

33	
As	
Arsenic	
74.92159	

Full name: Arsenicum Album
Other names: White oxide of arsenic, Arsenic trioxide

The homeopathic remedy Arsenicum is made from the compound arsenic trioxide. Arsenic trioxide is a white, crystalline powder that occurs naturally in some minerals and ores.

USEFUL FOR:

ANXIETY: Tremendous anxiety with great restlessness. Panic attack after midnight. Despair of recovery. Health anxiety. Fastidious - likes order. Fear of germs and dirt. Needs company.

FOOD POISONING: Diarrhoea with vomiting. Watery vomiting until stomach empty then vomiting bile. Exhaustion.

FEVER: From Midnight to 2am. Restlessness, anxiety, chilliness, craves warmth and thirsty for small sips.

FLU: Extreme weakness, Craves warmth. Exhaustion yet restlessness. Worse after midnight. Wants company and fears death.

HAYFEVER: Thin watery burning discharges. May have itching in nose, eyes or throat.

RESPIRATORY ISSUES: Very anxious and restless. Exhausted. Asthma attacks from midnight to 2am. Desires company. Symptoms helped by sitting up and hindered by lying down.

STOMACH: Gastritis with extreme burning. Indigestion with burning sensation. Desire to sip water or warm drinks. Helped by drinking milk. Diarrhoea with offensive watery stools.

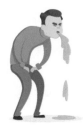

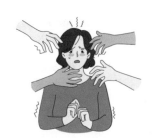

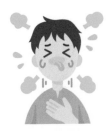

Belladonna
Sudden inflammation, high fevers, sore throats

KEY SYMPTOMS:

- Sudden, intense, violent onset
- Redness and heat
- Inflammations
- Dilated pupils
- Throbbing pains
- Symptoms come and go like a storm
- Hot head
- Icy cold hands and feet
- Intense pain
- Thirstless - may crave lemonade
- Rapid pulse
- Hot flushes
- Convulsions, twitches or jerking

dry, hot, red skin flushed face

sudden intense symptoms that come and go like a storm

dilated pupils

lack of thirst, may crave lemonade

delirium

MENTAL SYMPTOMS
'Angel when well devil when sick'
Fever terrors or delirium
Rage, anger, biting

EVENT THAT CAUSED SYMPTOMS:
Head getting wet
Walking in a draft or wind
Ill effects of haircut
Sunstroke

haircut

sunstroke

< touch

> pressure

Hindered by:
Afternoon
Light
Noise
Motion or being jarred
Touch

Helped by:
Cold
Pressure
Crying or moaning
Eating
Lying propped up

Belladonna
Cheat sheet

Other names: Deadly nightshade, Atropa belladonna
Made from the plant Atropa belladonna, commonly known as deadly nightshade. It is a perennial herbaceous plant that belongs to the Solanaceae family. It is native to Europe, North Africa and Western Asia.

USESFUL FOR:
COUGHS: Tickling, short, dry cough. Worse at night.

EARS: Hot, sensitive, painful ears. Throbbing, tearing, stitching pain. Pain may spread down into the neck or face.

EYES: Pupils dilated. Conjunctivitis with lots of inflammation. Eyelids swollen and congested. Photophobia. Sensation as if eyes half closed.

FEMALE: Period pains. Hot, throbbing pains. Hindered by motion. Mainly right sided. Pains in ovaries which is worse before menses. Menopause - hot flashes.

FEVER: High dry fever. Dilated pupils. Fever terror or hallucinations. Child may not recognise the parent. Convulsions from fever. Hitting, biting, anger and rage. Lack of thirst - may crave lemonade.

HEADACHES AND MIGRAINES: Pulsating, throbbing, bursting. Fullness and pain, especially in forehead. Helped by resting the head, no noise, dark room. Useful for sunstroke.

MASTITIS: Often right sided. Red, painful and worse for jarring.

TEETHING: Red, hot, throbbing pain. May have dilated pupils.

THROAT: Sore throat, Scarlet fever, strep throat and tonsillitis. High fever. Redness, Throbbing pain, Lack of thirst. Hindered by swallowing.

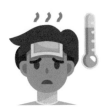

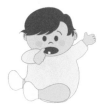

Bellis Perennis
A deeper acting Arnica - for deep tissue injuries

KEY SYMPTOMS:

- Useful for when Arnica fails or when bumps remain after a bruise
- Injuries, blows, strains with great soreness
- Septic wounds
- Post surgery
- Post childbirth
- Fall on the coccyx
- Tumours or cysts from injury
- Throbbing pain
- Squeezing pain
- Acrid pus
- Abscesses of abdomen/pelvic area
- Boils and swelling
- Varicose veins

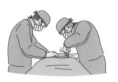

use post surgery

soreness & deep bruising

acrid pus

when bumps remain after a bruise

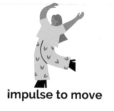

impulse to move

MENTAL SYMPTOMS
Impulse to move

EVENT THAT CAUSED SYMPTOMS:
Surgery such as post c-section
Injury to soft tissue
From hard physical work such as gardening
Childbirth

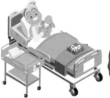

childbirth or c-section

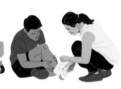

injury to soft tissue

< cold drinks

> cold application

Hindered by:
Touch
Cold baths/drinks
Becoming chilled when hot
Left side

Helped by:
Cold application
Continuous motion

HELP! Bellis Perennis
Cheat sheet

Other names: English daisy
Part of the 'tough daisy family (includes other first aid remedies like Arnica and Calendula). Although many other related plants are also called daisy, Bellis perennis is often considered the archetypal species.

USEFUL FOR:

ABSCESSES: Acrid pus. Abscesses especially of abdomen and pelvic area.

ACCIDENTS AND INJURIES: Injuries to deeper tissues. Sprains and bruises. Soreness and swelling. Tumours or cysts from injuries.

BREASTS: Injuries to breasts. Use post mammogram.

JOINT PAINS: Sore and bruised sensation. Aching.

SKIN: Boils. Acrid pus. Bruises especially when bumps remain after a bruise..

POST SURGERY AND POST LABOUR: To help speed up healing. Helps with soreness. Relieves pain and bleeding after childbirth. Tones uterus.

VARICOSE VEINS: With bruised sore feeling.

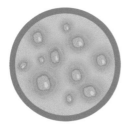
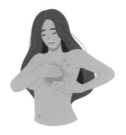
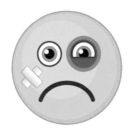

Bryonia
Dry painful coughs, flu, migraines

KEY SYMPTOMS:
- Slow onset Inflammation
- Dryness
- Dry lips
- Every movement hurts
- Aching bones and joints
- Must lie motionless
- Holds onto affected part
- Bursting and stitching pains
- Splitting headache
- Dry, hacking, painful coughs
- Constipation due to large, dry stools
- Thirsty - drinks in glugs

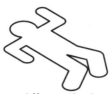

must lie motionless like a corpse

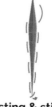

bursting & stitching pains

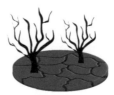

dryness

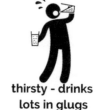

thirsty - drinks lots in glugs

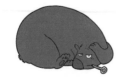

bear with sore head desires solitude

MENTAL SYMPTOMS
Bear with a sore head
Desires solitude
Money or work worries
May say 'I want to go home'

EVENT THAT CAUSED SYMPTOMS:
Anger
Fright
Alcohol

anger

alcohol

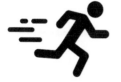

< movement

> pressure

Hindered by:
Any movement
Stooping
On rising
Coughing
Deep breathing
Exertion

Helped by:
Pressure
Resting in bed
Lying on painful part
Cool open air
Quiet
Heat to the painful area

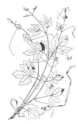

Bryonia
Cheat sheet

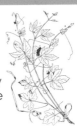

Full name: Bryonia Alba
Other names: Wild hops, white bryony
The homeopathic remedy Bryonia is made from the plant Bryonia alba, commonly known as white bryony or wild hops. Bryonia alba is a climbing, flowering vine native to Europe and parts of Asia.

USEFUL FOR:

COUGHS AND RESPIRATORY ISSUES: Pneumonia. Irritating, dry cough. Coughing fits. Pain on coughing - may hold chest on coughing to stop any movement. Helped by pressure to painful part. Intense thirst, dry lips.

FLU: Slow onset. Dryness -dry lips. Every movement hurts. Aching bones and joints. Must lie motionless. Can have extreme exhaustion, Thirsty - drinks in glugs. Wants to be alone.

HEADACHES AND MIGRAINES: Bursting intense pain behind the eyeballs, worse for any movement, even movement of the eyes. Left sided. Dizziness when turning in bed. Helped by pressure and cold application.

JOINTS: Swelling with stitching pain. Better for tight bandage and resting on the painful part.

MASTITIS: Gradual onset. Sore and hard breasts. Flu like symptoms.

STOMACH: Gastritis. Nausea and vomiting after eating. Thirsty - drinks in glugs. Constipation with dryness of rectum. Stools are dry and hard. Sensation of a stone in the stomach. Indigestion.

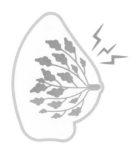

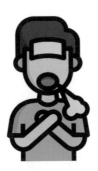

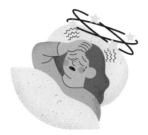

Calc Carb
Number 1 'constitutional' remedy for infants

KEY SYMPTOMS:
- Babies prone to frequent infections
- Chubby 'chunky monkey'
- Delayed milestones
- May have cradle cap
- Nightmares
- Sweats easily - may be sour
- Teething issues
- Fontanelles slow to close
- Constipation but actually feels happy for it
- Craves sweets and eggs
- Thick yellow bland discharges
- Swollen glands

frequent infections

sweaty

'buddha' babies

cradle cap

fearful

MENTAL SYMPTOMS
Fearful and anxious
Fear of the dark
Fear of dogs, small insects
Likes to observe before doing

EVENT THAT CAUSED SYMPTOMS:
Physical exertion
Mental exertion
Rudeness from others
Losing money/job

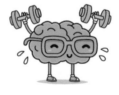

mental exertion

rudeness

< milk

> dry climate

Hindered by:
Bathing
Pressure of clothes
Milk
Teething

Helped by:
Dry climate
Dry weather
Lying on back/painful side

Calc Carb
Cheat sheet

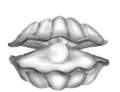

Full name: Calcarea Carbonica
Other names: Oyster shell, Calcium carbonate, Impure carbonate of lime
Calcium carbonate is a common compound which can be found in various forms including lime, chalk and marble. The homeopathic remedy is made from thick oyster shells.

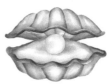

USEFUL FOR:

EARS: Enlarged glands. Cracking or throbbing in ears. Pulsating pain.

INSOMNIA: Night terrors. Nightmares in children, can wake up screaming. Dreams of monsters. Anxious thoughts arouses from light sleep. Insomnia due to worry.

RESPIRATORY ISSUES: Colds. Shortness of breath. Painless hoarseness. Suffocating spells. Dry nostrils. Takes cold at every change of weather.

STOMACH: Large and hard. Distension. Frequent sour belching. Chalky, grey or green stools. Stools hard at first and then liquid. Constipation in babies.

TEETHING: Difficult and slow dentition.

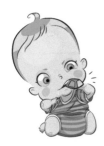

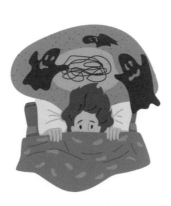

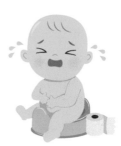

Calc Phos
Bone health, growing pains

KEY SYMPTOMS:

- Soft, thin and brittle bones
- Broken bones - promotes healing
- Osteoporosis
- Sensation of crawling or numbness
- Growing pains
- Enlarged tonsils
- Colic after feeding
- Craves smoked meats
- Backache with menses
- Rickets
- Baby refuses breastmilk
- Cold sensation in ears
- Headaches in school children

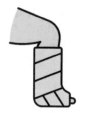
broken bones

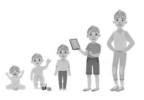
growing pains

craves smoked meats

weak bones

temper tantrums

MENTAL SYMPTOMS
Temper tantrums
Obstinate
Moaning
Difficult to please
Desire to travel

EVENT THAT CAUSED SYMPTOMS:
Bad news
Grief
Disappointed love
Overgrowth
Overstudy

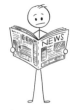
bad news

overstudy

< teething   **> summer**

Hindered by:
Teething
Puberty
Mental exertion
Loss of fluids
Artificial lights
Getting wet in rain

Helped by:
Summer
Warm, dry atmosphere
Lying down

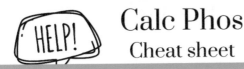

Calc Phos
Cheat sheet

Full name: Calcarea Phosphorica
Other names: Calcium phosphate,
Phosphate of lime, Tricalcic phosphate
Calc phos is made by dropping dilute phosphoric acid into lime water. Calc phos is also available as a 'tissue salt' which, although made in line with homeopathic principles (albeit to a less diluted level), still contains a material dose so works on a more physical level. The homeopathic remedy can work on a physical and mental level.

USEFUL FOR:

BONES: Growing pains. Rickets. Non-union of bones. Delayed healing of bones. Weak bones or bones slow to heal. Brittle bones. Osteoporosis. Curvature of the spine.

HEADACHES: Headaches in school children especially near puberty. May have diarrhoea.

STOMACH: Colic especially in babies or children after feeding. Babies who refuse to breast feed. Weak digestion. Flatulence.

TEETHING: Delayed dentition. Teeth decay easily.

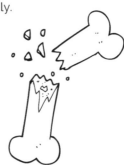

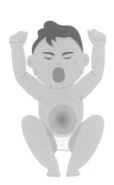

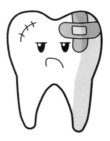

Calendula
The homeopathic antiseptic, wounds

KEY SYMPTOMS:

- Wounds, burns and ulcers
- Rawness
- Inflammation
- Excessive pain
- Swelling
- Whitish pus oozing from a closed wound
- Speeds up healing
- Post childbirth
- Post surgery
- Varicose veins
- Nappy rash

support wound healing   **pus from a closed wound**

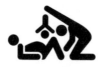

post childbirth healing   **post surgery healing**

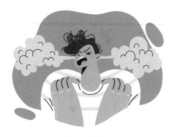

irritable

MENTAL SYMPTOMS

Irritable
Fearful

EVENT THAT CAUSED SYMPTOMS:

Burns, cuts, punctures, stabs, wounds, surgery

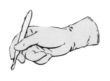

surgery   **wounds**

< heavy cloudy weather   **> warmth**

Hindered by:
Heavy, cloudy weather
Evening

Helped by:
Walking about
Warmth
Lying still

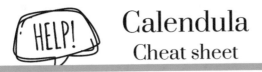

Calendula
Cheat sheet

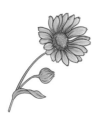

Full name: Calendula Officinalis
Other names: Pot marigold
Part of the 'tough daisy family.' Calendula can be found growing in barren soils. They are 'tough' and can survive harsh conditions. Calendula is known best as a tincture for the topical treatment of injuries.

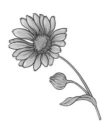

USES:
- Can be given as a homeopathic potentised remedy or also available as a cream or tincture.
- Promotes healing, reduces inflammation, stops and clears infection.
- Make sure any cuts are clean, with all debris removed, as calendula can cause fast healing, and may heal over dirt, foreign bodies etc.
- Use of tincture: 10/15 drops in small glass of cooled, boiled (or sterile) water for bathing/cleaning wounds. If it stings, it can be diluted more.
- Childbirth: Useful after childbirth when used to wash perineum.
- Nappy rash: Useful to sooth inflamed skin.

'It is the best herbal wound dressing and antiseptic that I know. Alack and alas! that so few, even keen homeopaths, appreciate its value as such...Calendula is wonderful for wounds with or without loss of substance, with sharp cutting pains, redness, rawness and sometimes stinging pain during febrile heat - then it acts like magic and promotes rapid healing.'
Dorothy Shepherd

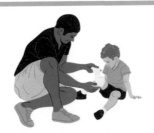

Candida Albicans
Homeopathic anti-fungal

KEY SYMPTOMS:
- Oral thrush
- Vaginal thrush
- Candidiasis
- Leucorrhea
- Vaginitis
- Flatulence
- Indigestion
- Bloated abdomen
- Loud rumbling in abdomen when lying down
- Gas

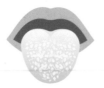

oral thrush

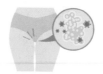

vaginal thrush

flatulence

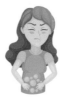

rumbling in tummy

Candida Albicans
Homeopathic anti-fungal

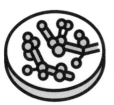
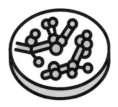

Other names: Thrush fungus
Candida Albicans is a homeopathic remedy
made from the fungus Candida Albicans.
Homeopathic remedies made out of
bacteria, fungi and other diseases, are called
'nosodes.'

Candida Albicans tends to be
prescribed therapeutically so
accompanying symptoms, event that
caused complaint and helped or
hindered are not generally taken into
account when deciding whether to give
this remedy.

DOSING

Follow regular
homeopathic dosing
principles. If frequent
dosing is needed then
add one pellet to a
bottle of water - one sip
equals one dose (and
this one sip is equivalent
to one pill).

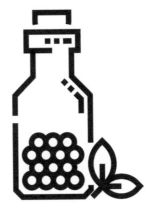

Cantharis
Burns, burning pains, cystitis

KEY SYMPTOMS:
- Burning pains
- Cutting pains
- Smarting pains
- Blisters
- Burning before, during and after urination
- Blood in urine
- Intense diarrhoea with bleeding
- Throat/larynx as if on fire
- Burning unquenchable thirst

burning pains

blisters

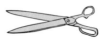

cutting pains

blood in urine

irritable

MENTAL SYMPTOMS
Angry
Irritable
Restlessness

EVENT THAT CAUSED SYMPTOMS:
Burns
Sunburn

burns

sunburns

< sound of water

> cold applications

Hindered by:
Urinating
Touch
Sound of water
Night
Coffee

Helped by:
Cold applications

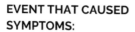

HELP!

Cantharis
Cheat sheet

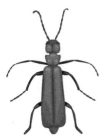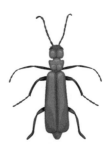

Full name: Cantharis Vesicatoria
Other names: Spanish fly, Lytta vesicator
Cantharis is a homeopathic remedy made from the substance known as Spanish fly, which is a species of blister beetle. They are found in North America, Europe and Asia. Blister beetles contain a toxic substance called cantharidin, which can cause irritation and blistering of the skin and mucus membranes.

USEFUL FOR:

BLADDER: Acute severe cystitis. Feels like constantly needs to urinate. Burning and cutting pains before, during and after urination. Intense burning in urethra. Violent and cutting pains in neck of bladder. May have blood in urine. Dribbling urine.

SKIN ISSUES INCLUDING BURNS: Rawness and smarting burns. Helped by cold applications. Sunburn. Blisters. Eruptions which burn when touched.

STOMACH: Burning stools. Bloody stools. Shuddering after passing stools.

THROAT: Difficulty swallowing, burning pain in mouth.

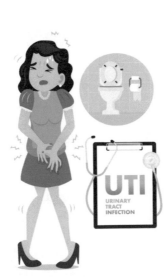
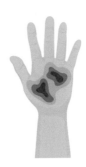

Capsicum
Ear infections, homesickness

KEY SYMPTOMS:

- Burning pains
- Red cheeks and face but cold
- Swelling and pain behind ears
- Thirsty but drinking causes shuddering
- Greenish tongue
- Bleeding from hemorrhoids
- Pain and dryness in throat
- Sensation of soreness and constriction
- History of repeated strep infections

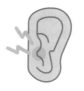

ear infections

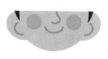

red cheeks

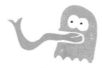

green tongue

history of strep infections

delirium

MENTAL SYMPTOMS

Delirium
Homesickness
Irritable

EVENT THAT CAUSED SYMPTOMS:

Homesickness

homesickness

< cold air

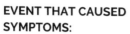

> heat

Hindered by:
Slight draft
Cold air
Dampness
After eating
Bathing

Helped by:
Continued motion
Heat
While eating

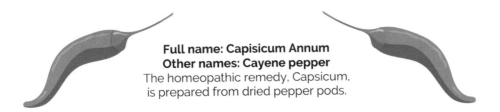

Capisicum
Cheat sheet

HELP!

Full name: Capisicum Annum
Other names: Cayene pepper
The homeopathic remedy, Capsicum,
is prepared from dried pepper pods.

USEFUL FOR:

EARS: Swelling and pain. Inflammation of mastoid. Hot ears. Burning and stinging in ears. Inflammation of Eustachian tube with much pain. Thirsty which may cause shuddering.

MIND: Homesickness with red cheeks and insomnia.

RECTUM: Hemorrhoids with bleeding. Sore anus. Bloody mucus. Burning. Small, hot, burning stools.

THROAT: Pain and dryness in throat. Throat feels constricted with urge to swallow.

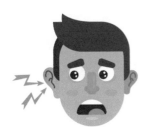

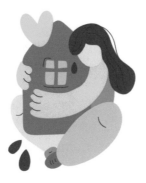

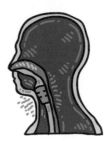

Carbo Veg
'The Corpse Reviver', collapse, digestive issues

KEY SYMPTOMS:
- Faint pulse
- Blue fingertips
- Feet icy cold up to the knees
- Head hot, cold breath and body
- Haemorrhage (anywhere)
- Hungry for air
- Can't tolerate tight clothing
- Violent spasmodic cough
- Wants to be fanned
- Abdomen bloated with gas
- Indigestion
- Plenty of belching
- Blue around mouth

bloated - can't tolerate tight clothing

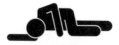

collapse

faint pulse

belching

low vitality

MENTAL SYMPTOMS
Low vitality
Exhaustion

EVENT THAT CAUSED SYMPTOMS:
Shock - post operation, blood loss
Prolonged nursing
Exhausting disease

blood loss

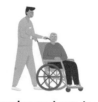

prolonged nursing

< pressure of clothes

> belching

Hindered by:
Warmth
Rich foods
Old age
Over lifting
Pressure of clothes
Extreme weather temps
Wind on head

Helped by:
Elevating the feet
Belching
Cool air - fanning
Sitting up

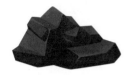 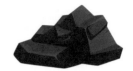

Carbo Veg
Cheat sheet

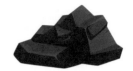

Full name: Carbo Vegetabilis
Other names: Vegetable charcoal
This remedy is made from vegetable charcoal which is a result of wood being burned in an inadequate supply of oxygen.

USEFUL FOR:

COLLAPSE: Lack of reaction. Blueness and decomposition. Almost lifeless. Known as 'the corpse reviver.'

COUGHS AND RESPIRATORY ISSUES: Must be fanned. Quick, short and laborious breathing. Cough with burning in chest. Blue face. Wheezing and rattling of mucus in chest. Thick, sticky and yellow expectoration. Asthma in the elderly.

HEMORRHAGE: Dark blood days after surgery. Stagnated blood.

STOMACH: Indigestion. Distended stomach. Flatulence. Colic. Helped by passing wind and belching. Cannot stand tight clothing around waist. Nausea and vomiting. Food poisoning caused by rotten fish or meat.

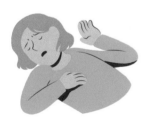

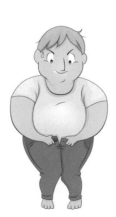

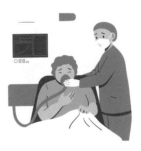

Caulophyllum
Childbirth, joint pains

KEY SYMPTOMS:
- False labour pains for days
- Weak, irregular or spasmodic contractions
- Sharp, shooting or radiating pain yet ineffective contractions
- Cervix that is slow to dilate
- Nervous exhaustion, fatigue or emotional stress during labour
- Chilliness, shivering or trembly
- Rheumatic remedy especially for small joints
- May have large thirst

weak contractions

prolonged or slow labour

rheumatism in small joints

false labour

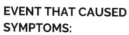

nervous

MENTAL SYMPTOMS
Nervous
Fretful

EVENT THAT CAUSED SYMPTOMS:
Childbirth
Miscarriages

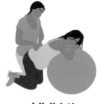

childbirth

miscarriage

< open air

Hindered by:
Pregnancy
Suppressed menses
Open air
Coffee

Helped by:
None noted

Caulophyllum
Cheat sheet

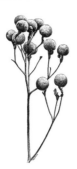
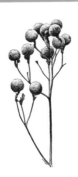

Full name: Caulophyllum Thalictroides
Other names: Blue cohosh, Squaw root
This remedy is made from the root of the blue cohosh plant. The plant is native to Eastern North America and has a long history of use by indigenous people for a variety of medicinal purposes, including aiding in childbirth.

USEFUL FOR:

CHILDBIRTH: Weak, irregular or spasmodic contractions. False labour for days. Prolonged or slow labour with weak or irregular contractions. Contractions may be in lower half of uterus. Sharp, shooting or radiating pain yet ineffective contractions. Cervix that is slow to dilate. Nervous exhaustion, fatigue or emotional stress during labour. General muscle weakness or a lack of strength during labour. Chilliness, shivering, irritability or trembly. May have large thirst. Worse for open air.

JOINT PAINS: Rheumatism of small joints. Sore nodes on finger joints. Aching in wrists.

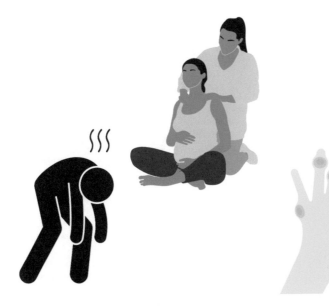

Causticum
Grief, joints, urinary issues, coughs

KEY SYMPTOMS:

- Loss of muscular strength
- Paralysis of parts or organs (including facial)
- Urinary incontinence on coughing
- Falls easily
- Tightness in chest
- Hollow, dry, incessant cough
- Weakness from longstanding grief or disease
- Convulsions, cramps, restlessness and twitching
- Stiffness and contracting of joints and limbs
- Raw, burning, sore and tender pains
- Headache - sensation as if empty space between skull and brain
- Warts

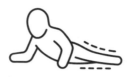
paralysis

burning pains

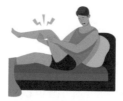
restlessness

urinary incontinence

intolerance of injustice

MENTAL SYMPTOMS
Intolerance of injustice
Anxiety of conscience
Oversympathetic

EVENT THAT CAUSED SYMPTOMS:
Burns and scalds
Grief
Nightwatching

burns

nightwatching

< fine weather

> cold drinks

Hindered by:
Clear fine weather
Dry cold air
Winds, drafts
Darkness
After stool
Coffee

Helped by:
Cold drinks
Damp wet weather
Washing

Causticum
Cheat sheet

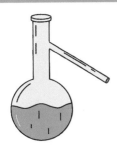

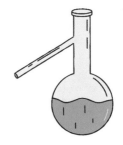

Other names: Caustic potash, Potassium hydrate
This remedy is made by distilling a mixture of slaked lime and a solution of potassium sulphate.

USEFUL FOR:

ANXIETY: Feels as if she had committed a crime. Timid and nervous. Oversensitive children who do not want to go to bed alone.

BLADDER: Paralysis of bladder. Involuntary passing of urination on coughing. Urine dribbles. Burning in urethra when urinating. Retention of urine after surgery or childbirth.

BURNS: Never been well since a burn. Old burns that do not heal.

COUGHS AND RESPIRATORY ISSUES: Hollow, hard and dry cough. Cough from tickling of larynx. Oppressive breathing worse for talking or walking. Wandering chest pains. Cannot cough deeply enough.

JOINTS: Contracted tendons. Rheumatism. Paralysis. Twisting and jerking in limbs. Burning in joints. Unsteady walking and easily falling. Restless legs at night. Pain in back worse for coughing.

THROAT: Lost voice of singers. Laryngitis.

WARTS: Bleed easily. Large warts. May be flat, fleshy or hard. Painful.

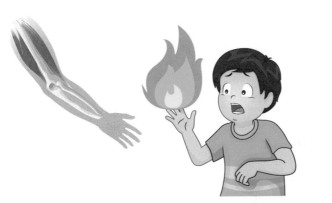

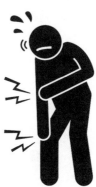

Chamomilla
Pain, teething, ear infections, colic

KEY SYMPTOMS:
- Beside oneself with pain
- Oversensitivity
- Hot and sweaty
- Colicky pains
- Teething
- Belching like bad eggs
- Green diarrhoea
- Flushed face - may have one red cheek
- Does not want to be looked at or touched

unbearable pain

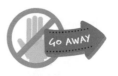

aversion to being looked at or touched

flushed face (can be one sided)

hot & sweaty

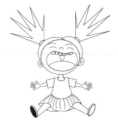

impossible to please

MENTAL SYMPTOMS
Inconsolable anger
Impossible to please - refuses what was requested
Demands to be carried

EVENT THAT CAUSED SYMPTOMS:
Excitement
Anger
Teething
Coffee
Alcohol

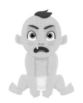

teething

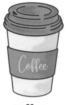

coffee

< 9pm - midnight

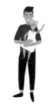

> being carried

Hindered by:
9pm - midnight
Cold air
Cold damp
Being looked at/touched

Helped by:
Being carried
Being uncovered

HELP! Chamomilla
Cheat sheet

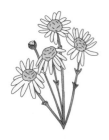
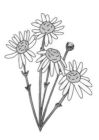

Full name: Chamomilla Vulgaris
Other names: German Chamomile,
Chamomile matricaria
This remedy is made from the dried flowers of the chamomile plant which grows especially well in sandy areas of Europe. It is one of the 'angriest' homeopathic remedies that there is.

USEFUL FOR:
COLIC: Inconsolable, arches back, cries angrily.

EAR INFECTION: Earache with soreness, swelling and heat which makes the individual feel frantic. Roaring in ears as if rushing water. Ears sensitive to touch. Wakes at night crying - inconsolable, angry and must be carried. Doesn't want to be touched or looked at. Sensitive to the wind.

FEVER: Thirsty, restless and irritable. Sweaty head.

INSOMNIA: Restless sleep, wakes often. Weeping in sleep.

PAINS: Unbearable pain that can bring on anger. Beside oneself with pain. May swear and scream in pain.

TEETHING: Irritable, sore gums, may have green diarrhoea.

STOMACH: Diarrhoea during teething. Stool with 'rotten egg' odour. Stools like cut grass or spinach. Belching like bad eggs. Thirsty for cold drinks. Colic.

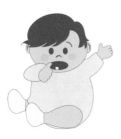
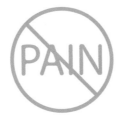
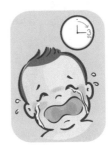

Chelidonium
Homeopathic liver support

KEY SYMPTOMS:

- Liver support
- Liver pains going backwards
- Sharp aching pain on right hand side
- Skin may be yellow-grey
- Also good for neonatal jaundice
- Craving for sweets
- Itching skin
- Burning pain like stinging nettles
- May have red pimples
- Nausea and bilious vomiting with sick headaches

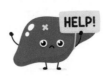

affinity to liver

itching - burning pain like stinging nettles

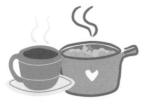

helped by hot food and drinks

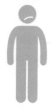

yellow or grey skin

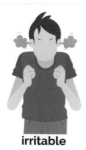

irritable

MENTAL SYMPTOMS
Cross and irritable'
Gets upset easily

EVENT THAT CAUSED SYMPTOMS:
Gallbladder obstruction

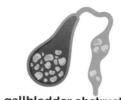

gallbladder obstruction

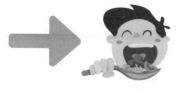

< right side   > after eating

Hindered by:
Right side
Coughing
Looking up
Change of weather'
4am and 4pm

Helped by:
After eating
Hot food
Lying on abdomen
Pressure

Chelidonium
Homeopathic liver support

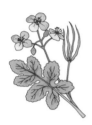
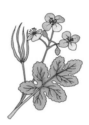

Full name: Chelidonium Majus
Other names: Greater Celadine
The homeopathic remedy Chelidonium is made from the plant commonly known as Greater Celandine, a herbaceous perennial plant belonging to the poppy family. It is native to Europe and parts of Asia but has also been naturalised in North America and other regions. It is closely allied to Lycopodium- when Lycopodium seems indicated but fails to act then Chelidonium should be considered.

USEFUL FOR:
- A major liver remedy with a keynote of sharp aching pains at the right scapula
- Yellowness and bilious complaints
- Gallbladder colic
- Bilious headaches - headaches over the right eye with a bad taste in the mouth
- Vomiting bile
- Irritability

DOSING

A great liver support remedy. Can take in a low potency (3 or 6c) daily for several weeks.

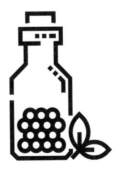

China
Exhaustion, weakness, collapse, loss of fluids

KEY SYMPTOMS:
- Exhaustion and debility due to loss of vital fluids (e.g. diarrhoea or blood)
- Hemorrhages including nosebleeds
- Poor circulation
- Headaches - throbbing, feels as if brain is floating in the skull
- Pale face, sunken eyes, dark rings around eyes
- Painless diarrhoea
- Ringing in ears
- Post operative gas pains
- Bloating - belching does not help
- Periodicity of symptoms.

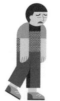

exhaustion & weakness

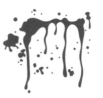

blood loss

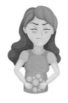

bloating

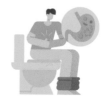

diarrhoea

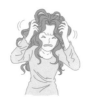

irritable and touchy

MENTAL SYMPTOMS
Irritable, sensitive and touchy
Clearness of mind in the evening

EVENT THAT CAUSED SYMPTOMS:
Loss of fluids
Blood loss
Food poisoning

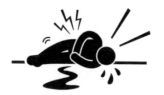

loss of fluids

food poisoning

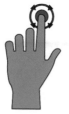

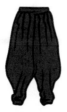

Hindered by:
Slightest touch
Loss of vital fluids
After eating
Impure water

Helped by:
Loose clothes
Hard pressure

< touch   > loose clothes

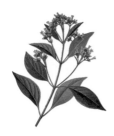

Full name: China Officinalis
Other names: Peruvian bark, Cinchona
The first substance that Hahnemann proved. Peruvian bark is an evergreen tree indigenous to South America but now found in India and parts of Asia. Quinine, a widely used treatment for malaria, is extracted from Peruvian bark.

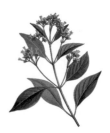

USEFUL FOR:

EXHAUSTION: Debility due to profuse discharges or loss of vital fluids. This remedy affects the blood helping improve circulation.

FOOD POISONING: Food poisoning especially from bad water, meat or fruit. Severe diarrhoea.

HEADACHES Intense throbbing of head. Congestive headaches.

RESPIRATORY ISSUES: Suffocative catarrh, rattling in lungs. Wants to be fanned but not too hard. Puffy, rattling breathing. Pneumonia after blood loss. Asthma worse in damp weather or after depletion.

STOMACH: Gas and bloating. Indigestion. Post surgery gas pains yet no relief when passes wind. Traveller's diarrhoea. Very sensitive to touch and pressure, especially around abdomen. Fermentation in the bowels especially after eating fruit. Flatulent colic.

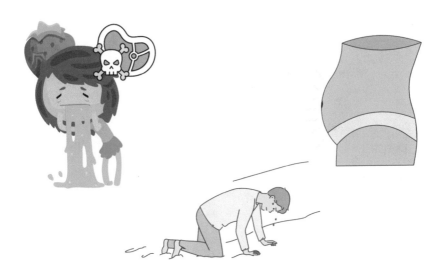

Cimicifuga
Hormonal issues. post natal depression, childbirth

KEY SYMPTOMS:

- Dark, profuse menses with a sensation of weight in uterus
- Pain across pelvis from hip to hip
- Displaced labour pains, weak contractions or slow labour
- Crampy pains
- Shooting, wandering pains which are like electric shocks
- Shooting pains in eye
- Extreme thirst
- Sighing
- Gnawing pain in stomach

painful, heavy periods

pain from hip to hip

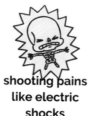

shooting pains like electric shocks

thirsty

as if black cloud over them

MENTAL SYMPTOMS

Depression as if a black cloud were sitting over them
Indifferent and apathetic
Feeling of impending doom
Aversion to communicate

EVENT THAT CAUSED SYMPTOMS:

Anxiety
Fright
Business failures
Childbirth

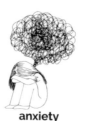

anxiety

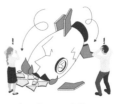

business failure

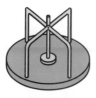

< motion

> eating

Hindered by:
Change of weather
Wine
Hormonal changes
Damp, cold air
Motion

Helped by:
Warm wraps
Open air
Pressure
Continued motion
Eating

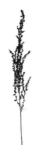
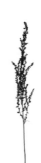

HELP! Cimicifuga
Cheat sheet

Full name: Cimicifuga Racemosa
Other names: Black Cohosh, Black snakeroot

Cimicifuga racemosa, also known as black cohosh. The plant is native to eastern North America and has been used by indigenous people for various medicinal purposes, including to treat menstrual irregularities and to aid in childbirth.

USEFUL FOR:

BACK PAIN: Stiffness and contraction in neck and back.

CHILDBIRTH: Physical symptoms similar to Caulophyllum. Pains like electric shocks. Contractions in lower half of uterus yet MOVE FROM SIDE TO SIDE or down into the hips and thighs. Sharp or spasmodic pains. Feels 'I can't carry on'. Cervix fails to dilate. Slow labour. Weak and ineffective contractions. Pains felt in hips, back or thighs. Talks incessantly. Sense of dread or fear (possibly previous bad experience). May be helped by lying on left side and open air.

FEMALE: Period pains. Pain that moves across pelvis from hip to hip. Profuse, dark and clotted menses. Pain in ovaries and breasts. Headaches in days leading up to period. Menopause - flushing and heat on top of head.

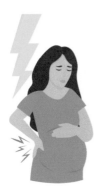
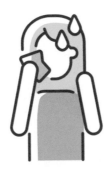
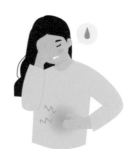

Cina
Worms, bedwetting

KEY SYMPTOMS:

- Number 1 remedy for worms
- Itchy bottom - may have spots and skin irritation
- Extreme sensitiveness of mind and body
- Nose picking and irritation
- Teething grinding during sleep
- Twitching and spasms
- Sour smell of body
- Ravenous hunger
- Stomach pains with twisting, cutting and pinching sensation
- Blue rings around eyes
- Bedwetting worse around full moon

pinworms

nose picking

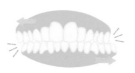

teeth grinding

bedwetting

angry child

MENTAL SYMPTOMS
Extreme anger - striking, screaming and biting
Impossible to please

EVENT THAT CAUSED SYMPTOMS:
Parasites

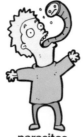
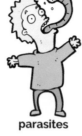

parasites

< full moon

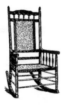

> rocking

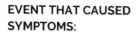

Hindered by:
Worms
During sleep
Touch
Full moon

Helped by:
Lying on abdomen
Rocking

Cina
Cheat sheet

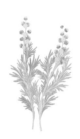

Full name: Cina Maritima
Other names: Wormseed. Artemesia,
Tartarian southernwood
Cina is a herb found mainly in Europe. Since
the time of Hippocrates it has been known
for its powerful anti-worm properties.

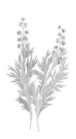

USEFUL FOR:
COUGHS: Whooping cough. Gagging in the morning. Violent recurring cough.

LIMBS: Twitching and jerking.

SLEEP: Grinds teeth at night during sleep. Night terrors of children. Cries and screams out and wakes frightened.

STOMACH: Ravenous hunger. Hunger after eating. Eats lots but doesn't gain weight. Vomiting.

WORMS: Itching of anus. Roundworms or threadworms. Children cannot tolerate having hair brushed. Irritable and angry children. Picks nose even in sleep.

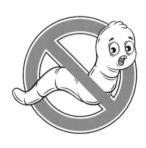

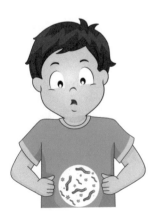

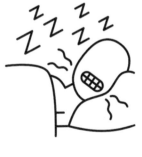

Cocculus
Nausea, vertigo, insomnia

KEY SYMPTOMS:

- Exhaustion
- Insomnia from disturbed sleep
- Vertigo - the world seems to spin
- Motion sickness
- Pregnancy sickness
- Metallic taste in mouth
- Thought of food creates nausea
- Weak lower back, worse during period
- Craving for beer
- Painful joints - knees crack on motion

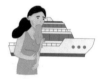

motion sickness

vertigo

morning sickness

exhaustion

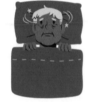

fearful of insomnia

MENTAL SYMPTOMS
Fearful of not getting enough sleep

EVENT THAT CAUSED SYMPTOMS:
Sleep loss
Nursing loved ones
Motion sickness

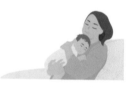

nursing / loss of sleep

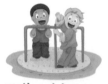

motion sickness

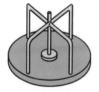

< motion

> warm room

Hindered by:
Loss of sleep (even an hour)
Alcohol
Motion
Nursing others

Helped by:
Lying quiet
Warm room

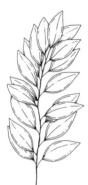

HELP!

Cocculus
Cheat sheet

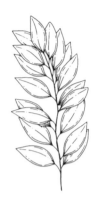

Full name: Cocculus Indicus
Other names: Indian Cockle, India berry.
This remedy is made from the Indian Cockle, a strong climbing tree found in parts of Malaysia and India which looks similar to a bay tree.

USEFUL FOR:

BACK PAIN: Weak, paralysed feeling in low back, worse menses.

INSOMNIA: Loss of sleep - from nursing a loved one, night watching or caring for a baby. Slightest loss of sleep aggravates. Sleep unrefreshing. Worries about not getting enough sleep. Sleep interrupted by starting and waking.

JET LAG: Eases overtiredness and disorientation. Helps to re-adjust.

JOINTS: Painful stiffness in joints. Trembling and pain in limbs. Knees crack on motion. Spasms of arms and legs.

NAUSEA/VERTIGO/TRAVEL SICKNESS: Seasickness and motion sickness. Feels as if may faint. Vertigo. Needs to lie down. Feels as if the world is spinning. Vomiting sour bitter.

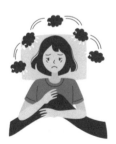

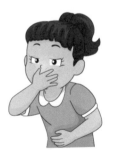

Colocynthis
Cramps, severe pains, colic

KEY SYMPTOMS:
- Pains better for bending double
- Colic - baby draws knees up to chest
- Pain helped by sharp pressure - so baby likes being carried over shoulder
- Cries out with pain
- Agonising cutting pains
- Boring pains in ovary
- Ovarian cysts
- Headache with sore scalp
- Sciatic pain which is helped by pressure and heat
- Bitter taste in mouth
- Jelly like stools
- Vertigo when turning head to the left

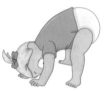

better for bending double

agonising colic

jelly like stools

likes being carried over shoulder

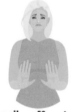

easily offended

MENTAL SYMPTOMS
Anger
Irritable
Joyless
Easily offended

EVENT THAT CAUSED SYMPTOMS:
Anger
After a cold
Grief

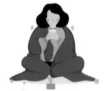

after a cold

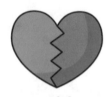

grief

< 4pm

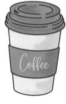

> coffee

Hindered by:
Lying on painless side
4pm
Lying in bed

Helped by:
Bending double
Hard pressure
Motion
Lying on abdomen
Coffee
Warmth

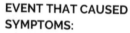

Colocynthis
Cheat sheet

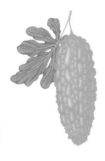
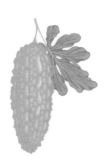

Other names: Bitter cucumber, Citrullus colocynthis, Bitter apple

The homeopathic remedy Colocynthis is made from the plant Citrullus colocynthis, commonly known as bitter cucumber. It is a desert plant found in the Mediterranean region and parts of Asia and Africa.

USEFUL FOR:

COLIC: Pains better for BENDING DOUBLE. Baby draws knees up to chest. Pain helped by sharp pressure so baby likes being carried over shoulder. Squirm and cry out with pain. May have slightly slimy nappies.

FEMALE: Boring pain in ovary. Ovarian cysts. Sharp pains before period.

STOMACH: Agonising cutting pain causing person to bend over double. Intestines feel as if they are being squeezed. Burning pain in anus. Violent cutting and tearing pains. Cramps in stomach at night. May even vomit from pain. Jelly like stools. Passing stools gives immediate relief. Pain worse for eating or drinking. Helped by motion such as twisting and wriggling around.

VERTIGO: Vertigo when turning head to lie on the left hand side of body.

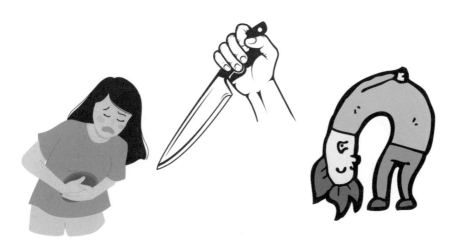

Dolichos
Itching, liver issues, constipation, hemorrhoids

KEY SYMPTOMS:
- Affinity to skin and liver
- Intense itching without eruptions
- Intolerable itching in pregnancy which is worse at night
- Itching prevents sleep
- No relief from itching
- Senile pruritus
- Constipation with itching
- Hemorrhoids with burning sensation
- Parasites including pinworms
- Bedwetting
- Bloated abdomen
- Taste of blood in the mouth
- Sore throat - as if vertical splinter

itching with no eruptions

constipation with itching

affinity to liver

sore throat as if vertical splinter

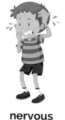

nervous

MENTAL SYMPTOMS
Nervousness

EVENT THAT CAUSED SYMPTOMS:
Getting feet wet

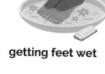

getting feet wet

< scratching   > cold applications

Hindered by:
Night
Scratching
Right side
Warmth

Helped by:
Cold applications
Lying on right

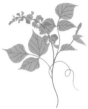

HELP! Dolichos
Cheat sheet

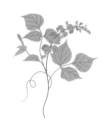

Full name: Dolichos Pruriens
Other names: Cowhage,
Mucuna pruriens, Cow-itch
This plant is a tropical legume native to India and other parts of South East Asia. It is a climbing shrub with distinctive velvety bean pods containing seeds covered in irritating hairs.

USEFUL FOR:

CONSTIPATION: Constipation with intense itching. Constipation during pregnancy or during teething. White stools. Pain in anus while passing stool.

HEMORRHOIDS: Hemorrhoids that are very painful, itchy and may be associated with a feeling of rawness and soreness in the anus. The itching is often intense and may become worse at night, disturbing sleep. Helped by cold applications and lying on abdomen.

ITCHING: Violent itching without any visible eruptions. Itching worse across shoulders, elbows, knees and hairy parts. Intolerable itching which is worse at night and prevents sleep. No relief from itching.

LIVER: Weak liver. Jaundice. Yellow spots or skin. Swelling of liver. Pain on left side. Liver issues with itching,

STOMACH: Worms and pinworms.

THROAT: Pain in throat as if a splinter embedded vertically.

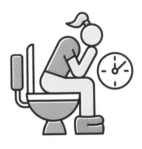

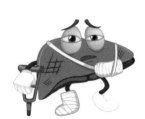

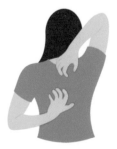

Drosera
Whooping cough, coughs

KEY SYMPTOMS:
- Spasmodic coughs
- Whooping cough
- Barking or choking coughs worse after midnight
- Fits of coughing
- Vomiting if cannot cough up phlegm
- Tightness or pains in chest
- Hoarse sore throat

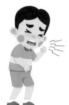

whooping cough

barking coughs

vomiting

hoarse sore throat

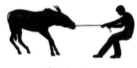

obstinate

MENTAL SYMPTOMS
Obstinate
Angry and irritable
Anxiety when alone

EVENT THAT CAUSED SYMPTOMS:
Cough after measles
Whooping cough

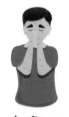

cough after measles

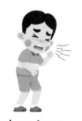

whooping cough

< after midnight

> pressure

Hindered by:
After midnight
Lying down
Talking
During rest

Helped by:
Pressure
Open air
Motion
Remaining quiet

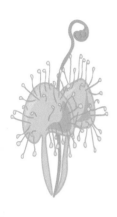
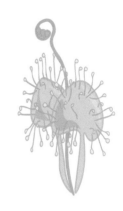

Full name: Drosera Rotunifolia
Other names: Round-leaved sundew,
Drosera longifolia

The homeopathic remedy Drosera is made from the sundew plant. Sundew is a small, carnivorous plant that is native to temperate and subarctic regions of North America, Europe and Asia.

The sundew plant is known for its distinctive appearance, with tiny, sticky, glandular hairs on its leaves that secrete a substance that traps and digests small insects. The plant uses this mechanism to supplement its nutrient intake, as it often grows in nutrient-poor soil.

USEFUL FOR:

COUGHS: Spasmodic cough that sounds like whooping cough. Coughing attacks in quick succession. Deep barking or choaking coughs. Fits of coughing. Coughs that are worse as soon as head hits the pillow.

RESPIRATORY ISSUES: Yellow expectorant. Retching. Oppressed breathing as if holding back the breath. Tightness of chest on coughing.

THROAT: Sore throat with rough, dry, scraping sensation. Hoarseness. Laryngitis.

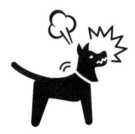
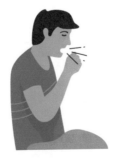
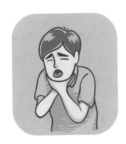

Eupatorium
Bone breaking pain, flu

KEY SYMPTOMS:
- Bone breaking pain
- Dry fever (no sweat)
- Muscles feel sore and bruised
- Hoarseness and cough with soreness in chest
- Headaches with soreness of eyeballs
- Thirsty for cold drinks (but may shudder or vomit after)
- Chilly but wants cold things
- Chill that starts at the small of the back
- Weakness

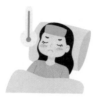

dry fever (no sweat)

bone breaking pains

bursting headache & sore eyes

chilly but wants cold things

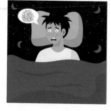

at night feels going out of one's mind

MENTAL SYMPTOMS
Extremely restless
Feels at night like going out of one's mind
Anxiety

EVENT THAT CAUSED SYMPTOMS:
'Ill effects of the ice house'

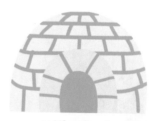

getting iced cold

< cold air

> getting on hands & knees

Hindered by:
Cold air
Periodically
Lying on part
7am to 9am
Coughing
Motion
Smell or sight of food

Helped by:
Vomiting bile
Lying on face
Sweating
Getting on hands and knees
Conversation

HELP! Eupatorium
Cheat sheet

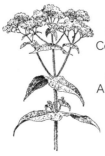

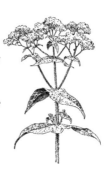

Full name: Eupatorium Perfoliatum
Other names: Boneset, Thoroughwort
Commonly known as Boneset, this remedy is made from the plant Eupatorium perfoliatum. This plant is native to North America and is known for its traditional use in herbal medicine for fever and colds.

USEFUL FOR:

COUGHS: Hoarseness and cough with soreness in chest. Cough better getting on hands and knees. Cough worse 2-4am.

FEVER: Weakness. Thirsty. Dry fever.

FLU: Bone breaking pain. Eyeballs ache and feel sore. Skin feels dry and sore. Chills in the back.

HEADACHES: Pain after lying down. Headaches with soreness of eyeballs. Sensation as if metal cap on head.

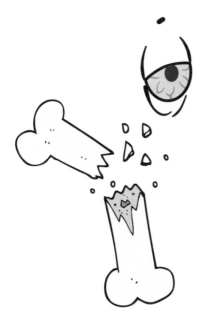

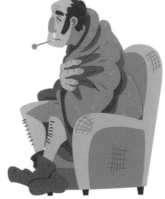

Euphrasia
Eye issues, hayfever, allergies, conjunctivitis

KEY SYMPTOMS:
- Watery burning eyes
- Bland nasal discharge
- As if sand in the eyes
- Frequent yawning when in open air
- Burning and swelling of the eyelids
- Hayfever
- Allergies
- Conjunctivitis
- Painful, late menses

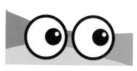
as if sand in eyes

bland nasal discharge

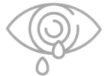
burning watery eyes

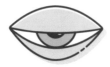
swelling of eyelids

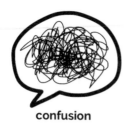
confusion

MENTAL SYMPTOMS
Aversion to answering
Confusion

EVENT THAT CAUSED SYMPTOMS:
Injuries
Measles
Flu

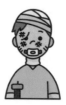
injuries

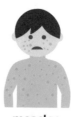
measles

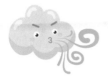
< wind

> open air

Hindered by:
Wind
Warmth
Sunlight
After sleep
Cold air
Lying down

Helped by:
Open air
Winking
Wiping eyes
Dark
Coffee
In bed

Euphrasia
Cheat sheet

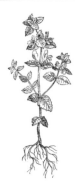
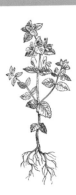

Full name: Euphrasia Officinalis
Other names: Eyebright
This small flowering plant is native to Europe and has been traditionally used in herbal medicine for various eye-related conditions.

USEFUL FOR:
ALLERGIES: Any allergic reaction where the eyes are involved or if the eye waters and swells.

EYES: As if sand in eyes. Eyes constantly water. Irritation extends to skin around the eyes and nose. Acrid, watery tears. Conjunctivitis. Thick yellow discharge. May want to blink frequently. Burning and swelling of the eyelids.

HAYFEVER: Acrid watery eyes, bland nasal discharge (opposite from Allium Cepa). Aversion to light.

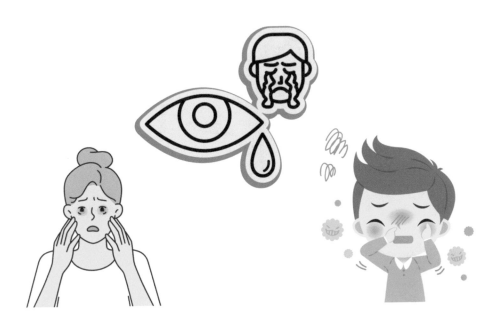

Ferrum Phos
When nothing seems to work...

KEY SYMPTOMS:

- 1st stage inflammation
- May take days to develop
- Stops colds descending to chest or ears
- Flushed face
- A 'mild belladonna'
- Heavy tired feeling
- Fevers
- Changeable mood
- In colds, eye may feel gritty
- Anaemia
- Any inflammations - tonsillitis, ear infections, headaches, bronchitis

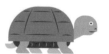

early stage! may take days to develop

in colds eyes may be gritty

stops colds descending to chest or ear

a 'mild belladonna'

> 'It is often difficult to prescribe Ferrum Phos because the type of case that requires this remedy is usually without localising or characterising symptoms. It is almost a diagnosis of exclusion. The typical case presents with high fever, often debilitating, and obvious inflammation of the effected part, be it throat, stomach, lungs etc. And yet despite the severity of the disease process, we find only general and vague symptoms which do not guide to any particular remedy '
> R. Morrison - Desktop Guide to Homeopathy

EVENT THAT CAUSED SYMPTOMS:
Suppressed sweat
Blood loss
Mechanical injuries

blood loss

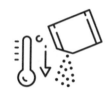

supressed sweat

< 4 to 6am

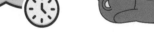

> lying down

Hindered by:
4-6am
Cold drinks

Helped by:
Lying down
Slow movement

HELP! Ferrum Phos
Cheat sheet

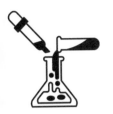
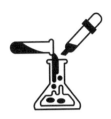

Full name: Ferrum Phosphorcium
Other names: Iron phosphate, Ferric phosphate

Ferrum phos is a remedy made from the chemical compound iron phosphate. Ferrum phos is also available as a 'tissue salt' which, although made in line with homeopathic principles (albeit to a less diluted level), still contains a material dose so works on a more physical level. The homeopathic remedy can work on a physical and mental level.

USEFUL FOR:

COLDS: helps to stop colds from descending to chest or ears.

EAR INFECTIONS: may be right sided. Few distinguishing symptoms. 'Nothing seems to work.'

FEVERS: Acute symptoms come on gradually, taking days to develop. No localising or individualising symptoms.

HEADACHES AND MIGRAINES: Flushes. Mild fever. Photophobia.

RESPIRATORY ISSUES: gradual onset. When nothing else seems to work.

SORE THROATS: Few distinguishing symptoms. 'Nothing seems to work.'

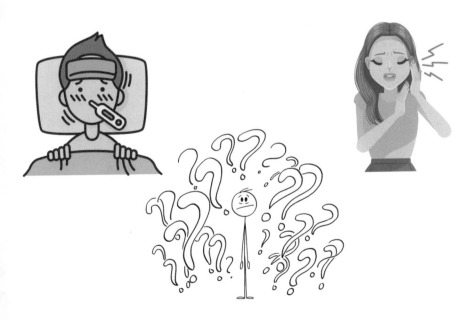

Gelsemium
Flu, anticipatory anxiety

KEY SYMPTOMS:
- Slow onset
- Trembly and chilly
- Heaviness
- Zombie like
- Tiredness
- Aching muscles
- Drooping of eyes
- Flu with shivering up and down the spine
- Dizzy when turning in bed
- Thirstlessness
- 'Never been well since' flu

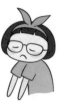

heaviness

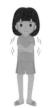

flu with shivers up and down the spine

droopy eyes

thirstless

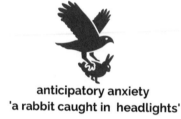

anticipatory anxiety
'a rabbit caught in headlights'

MENTAL SYMPTOMS
Anticipatory anxiety - like a rabbit caught in headlights

EVENT THAT CAUSED SYMPTOMS:
Fright
Bad news
Weather changing to warm after the cold of winter

bad news

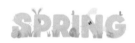

weather changing to warm

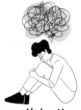

< anticipation

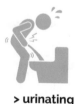

> urinating

Hindered by:
Movement
Thinking
Anticipation
Humid weather
Before a thunderstorm

Helped by:
Rest
Sweating
Urinating
Open air
Afternoon

HELP! Gelsemium
Cheat sheet

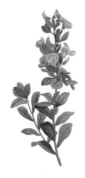
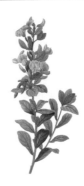

Full name: Gelsemium Sempervirens
Other names: Yellow jasmine
Gelsemium, also known as yellow jasmine, should not be confused with true jasmine. It is a beautiful climbing plant found in woodlands and along coastal areas in the Southern States of America.

USEFUL FOR:

ANXIETY: anticipatory anxiety - helps with the terror before a performance. Diarrhoea from fright or anticipation. Ailments from shock or fright.

FEVERS: Low grade fevers. Acute symptoms come on gradually, taking days to develop.

FLU: Extreme weakness with shivers up and down the spine. Heaviness with drooping eyelids. Thirstless. Complaints may start after bad news.

HEADACHES AND MIGRAINES: Vertigo. Dizzy when turning in bed. Headache beginning in the occiput or neck and radiating in the forehead. Headache helped by urinating. Heavy head as if it can be hardly lifted.

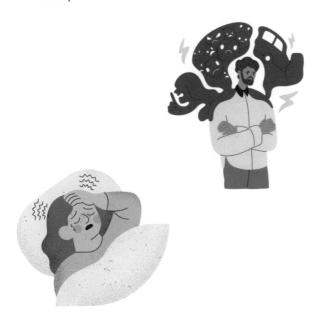
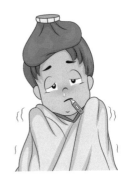

Hepar Sulph
Secondary inflammation, croup, boils, ear infections

KEY SYMPTOMS:

- Tendency to suppuration
- Boils and abscesses
- Catarrhal processes
- Thick yellow acrid ropey discharges
- Splinter like pains especially in the throat
- Painful ear infections with pus
- Sensitive to touch
- Coughs from exposure to cold, dry winds
- Profuse sweat
- Croupy coughs
- Deep cracks on hands and feet

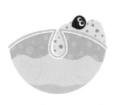

pus and suppuration

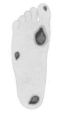

boils & abscesses

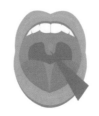

splinter like pains in throat

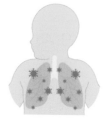

croupy coughs

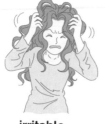

irritable

MENTAL SYMPTOMS
Sensitive to all impressions
Irritable
Impulsive

EVENT THAT CAUSED SYMPTOMS:
Cold, dry winds
Injuries
Suppressed eruptions
Abuse of mercury

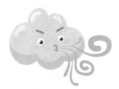

cold, dry wind

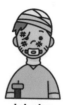

injuries

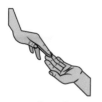

< touch

> damp weather

Hindered by:
Inhaling air
Cold air
Dry winds
Touch
Motion
Washing

Helped by:
Damp weather
Warmth
Wrapping head up
Pressure
After eating

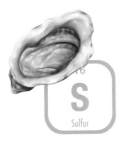

HELP!

Hepar Sulph
Cheat sheet

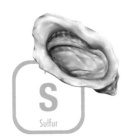

Full name: Hepar Sulphuris Calcareum
Other names: Calcium Sulphide
Prepared by burning the white interior of oyster shells with pure flowers of sulphur.

USEFUL FOR:

BOILS AND ABSCESSES: unhealthy skin. Ulcers with bloody discharges which smell like old cheese. Very sensitive skin. Wants to have skin wrapped up warmly.

COLDS: Thick, yellow, ropy discharges. Lots of catarrh. Sensitive to cold. Splinter like pains. Irritable. Sweaty.

COUGHS: Cough from exposure to cold or winds. Loose thick cough. Rattling cough. Suffocative attacks.

CROUP: Use if aconite fails.

EAR INFECTIONS: Splinter like pains. Ears sensitive to touch. Ear infections after being in a wind. Whizzing and throbbing. Discharge of pus from ears.

RESPIRATORY ISSUES: Breathing difficult. Worse when lying on the left side. Wheezing.

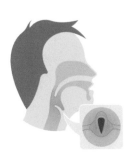

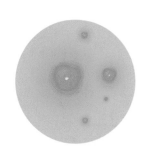

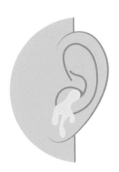

Histaminum
Homeopathic anti-histamine

KEY SYMPTOMS:
- Urticaria
- Allergic reactions
- Dryness of mucus membranes
- Redness and burning
- Red. itching papules
- Loss of taste
- Burning in the nose, throat and ears
- Vertigo
- Stinging pain in chest
- Edge of eyelids red
- Yellow secretions from eyes
- Conjunctivitis
- Insect bites
- Chicken pox - relieves itching
- Hayfever symptoms

urticaria

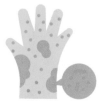

red itching papules

insect bites

dryness of mucus membranes

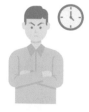

impatient

MENTAL SYMPTOMS
Impatient
Sensitive to slightest trifles

EVENT THAT CAUSED SYMPTOMS:
Allergic reactions
Bites

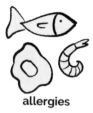

allergies

bites

< heat

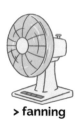

> fanning

Hindered by:
Heat
Movement

Helped by:
Pressure
Fanning

Histaminum
Cheat sheet

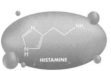

Other names: Histamine, Histamine hydrochloricum, Histaminum muriaticum
Histaminum is prepared from the chemical compound histamine, which is a biogenic amine involved in various physiological processes, including the immune response and allergic reactions.

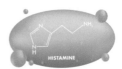

USEFUL FOR:

- All symptoms of the skin and mucus membranes in allergic types
- Dryness of mucus membranes
- Redness and burning of skin
- Red, itching papules which are helped by scratching
- Redness and heat of the face

DOSING

Follow regular homeopathic dosing principles. If frequent dosing is needed then add one pellet to a bottle of water - one sip equals one dose (and this one sip is equivalent to one pill).

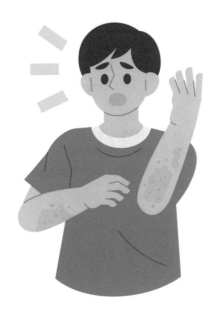

Hypericum
'Arnica of the nerves', crush injuries

KEY SYMPTOMS:

- Injuries to areas rich in nerves
- Nerve injury especially coccyx
- Crushed fingers especially tips
- Whiplash
- Excessive pain
- Tingling, burning and numbness
- Puncture wounds and bites
- Injured nerves from animal bites
- Anti-tetanus properties
- Post surgery
- Sharp shooting radiating pains
- Amputations – with severe neuralgia
- Paralysis from nerve injury
- Routinely given after root canal dental work

Crushed fingers, especially tips

puncture wounds

Injured nerves from animal bites

Nerve injuries especially fingers, toes & coccyx

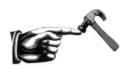

weak memory

MENTAL SYMPTOMS
Mistakes in speaking
Weak memory

EVENT THAT CAUSED SYMPTOMS:
Injections, gunshot, stab wounds, punctures, bites, stings
Surgery
Fright
Following a forceps delivery

surgery

stings

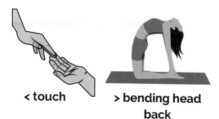

< touch   **> bending head back**

Hindered by:
Jar
Touch
Pressure

Helped by:
Bending head back
Rubbing

Hypericum
Cheat sheet

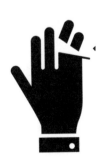

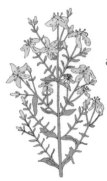

Full name: Hypericum Perforatum
Other names: St John's Wort
This plant can be found across temperate areas of Eurasia and has been introduced as an invasive weed to much of North and South America, as well as South Africa and Australia. It is used widely in herbal medicine, often for general depression, especially nervous depression.

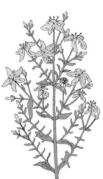

USEFUL FOR:

BACKACHE: Coccyx injury from fall. Pinched nerves in back. Violent sharp pain. Painfully sensitive spine.

BITES/STINGS: Infected wounds. Bites of animals and insects. Gunshot wounds.

INJURIES: Crush injuries. Any injury to the nerves especially fingers, toes and nails. Shooting pains from injured parts. Brain and spinal cord injuries. Tailbone pain from injuries. Lacerations with violent shooting pains. Infected wounds. Wounds are more tender than they look.

TEETH: Facial neuralgia and toothache. Helps speed up healing after dental work. Tingling, burning or numbness.

SURGERY: Relieves pain after surgery.

TETANUS: Reputed anti-tetanus properties.

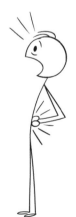

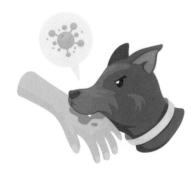

Ignatia
Acute grief, shock, disappointment, headaches

KEY SYMPTOMS:

- Grief, depression, disappointment and shock
- Suppressed menses especially from grief
- Cramps, twitching, tremors and tics
- Dry hacking spasmodic cough
- Sensation of lump in throat
- Palpitations especially at night
- Headaches like a nail driven into head
- May have 'air hunger' - sighing or yawning
- Empty feeling in the pit of stomach
- Colic and abdominal spasms especially at night

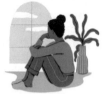

grief

air hunger such as sighing

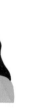

headache like a nail driven into head

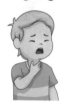

sensation like a lump in throat

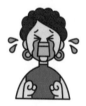

hysterical

MENTAL SYMPTOMS
Hysterical
Hypersensitivity
Unendurable grief
Alternating moods and erratic
Outbursts of sobbing or anger

EVENT THAT CAUSED SYMPTOMS:
Grief
Emotional shocks
Disappointment
Fright
Jealousy

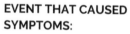

grief

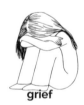

jealousy

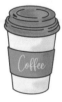

< coffee

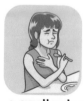

> swallowing

Hindered by:
Coffee
Tobacco

Helped by:
Eating
Swallowing
Deep breathing
Being alone

HELP!

Ignatia
Cheat sheet

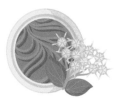 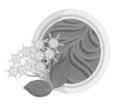

Full name: Ignatia Amara
Other names: St Ignatia's Bean,
Strychnos ignatia, Strychnos
multiflora, Faba indica
Made from the seeds of the plant
Strychnos ignatia This plant is native to
the Philippines and other South East
Asian countries. The seeds of the plant
contain a larger proportion of
strychnine than those of Nux Vomica,
which is from the same family.

USEFUL FOR:

COUGHS AND RESPIRATORY ISSUES: Constriction of chest. Dry, hacking and spasmodic coughs. Lots of sighing.

FEMALE: Menses which stop after grief. Threatened miscarriage after fright or grief.

HEADACHES AND MIGRAINES: Nervous headaches that come and go suddenly. Headache as if a nail being driven through the side.

HEART: Constriction of heart with anxiety and disposition to cry.

LIMBS: Spasms and cramps. Twitching of muscles. Spasmodic clenching of jaw.

MIND - ACUTE GRIEF: Suppressed or deep grief with long drawn out sighs. Hysteria. Changeable moods. Ailments from grief, emotional shocks and disappointments. Worse for consolation.

STOMACH: Abdominal spasms and cramps. Colic worse for coffee and sweets. Flatulent colic especially at night. Fullness and distension making breathing hard. Sinking feeling.

THROAT: Hysterical spasm of throat. Sensation as if lump in throat.

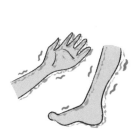 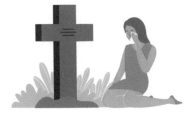 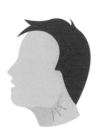

Ipecac
Flu, bronchitis, nausea

KEY SYMPTOMS:
- Nausea but vomiting does not ease
- Bronchitis - gasps for air
- Rattling cough without expectoration
- Whooping cough with retching or vomiting
- Bright red gushing hemorrhages with nausea
- Period pains with nausea
- Aversion to food
- Migraine with nausea
- Aching in the bones especially thighs and legs
- Cramps with nausea or cutting pain around navel

nausea but vomiting doesn't ease

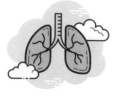

bronchitis - gasps for air

rattling cough

hemorrhages

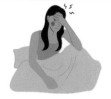

anxiety during fever

MENTAL SYMPTOMS
Anxiety during fever
Depression

EVENT THAT CAUSED SYMPTOMS:
Food poisoning
Vexation
Loss of blood
Rich food

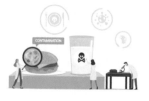

food poisoning

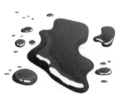

loss of blood

< morphine

> open air

Hindered by:
Drugs especially morphine
Overeating
Vomiting
Warmth
Damp
Warm, moist wind
Summer heat

Helped by:
Open air
Rest
Pressure
Closing eyes
Cold drinks

Ipecac
Cheat sheet

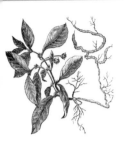

Full name: Ipecacuanha
Other names: Ipecac root, Cephaelis
ipecacuanha

Ipecacuanha, commonly known as Ipecac, is a homeopathic remedy made from the dried root of the plant Cephaelis ipecacuanha. The plant is native to South America, particularly Brazil.

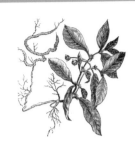

USEFUL FOR:

COUGHS: Violent and incessant cough. Whooping cough. Coughs with nausea and vomiting. Dry tickly cough. Rattling cough but with no expectoration.

HEADACHES AND MIGRAINES: Migraine headache with severe nausea and vomiting. Headache extends to face, teeth or root of tongue.

NAUSEA, VOMITING AND MORNING SICKNESS: Persistent nausea and vomiting. Profuse salivation. Constant desire to vomit. Disgust for food. Food poisoning.

RESPIRATORY ISSUES: Gasping for air. Shortness of breath. Wants open air. Loose, coarse rattle in chest without expectoration. Nausea.

STOMACH: Cramps with nausea and vomiting. Cutting pains which are worse around the naval. Griping pains. Colic in screaming and restless children. Diarrhoea especially in children due to overeating.

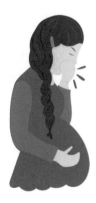

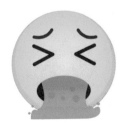

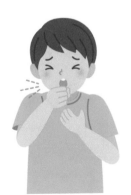

Kali Bich
Mucus, catarrh, colds, sinusitis. joint issues

KEY SYMPTOMS:

- Sinusitis - pressure and pain at bridge of nose
- Ropey or stringy mucus
- Thick, green, yellow or white discharges
- Post nasal drip
- Mucus difficult to cough up
- Loss of smell
- Headaches or migraines over eyebrows
- Wet asthma with stringy mucus
- Bladder issues including sensation of drop of urine remaining
- Rheumatism - arthritic pains which travel
- Cracking joints

sinusitis

stringy discharges

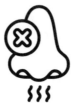

loss of smell

mucus in chest difficult to cough up

impatient

MENTAL SYMPTOMS
Impatience
Talks to oneself
Sadness

EVENT THAT CAUSED SYMPTOMS:
Overindulgence in beer and malt liquor

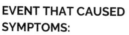

beer

malt liquor

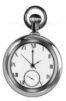

< 2-3am

> heat

Hindered by:
Suppressed catarrh
Alcohol
Beer
2-3am
Damp

Helped by:
Heat
Motion
Short sleep

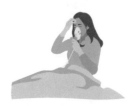

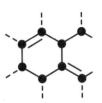 

Kali Bich
Cheat sheet

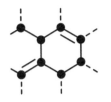

Full name: Kali Bichromicum
Other names: Potassium bichromate,
Potassium dichromate, Red Chromate
of Potash
Made from the chemical compound
potassium bichromate, a bright orange-
red, crystalline solid and is highly toxic in
its original form.

USEUL FOR:

COLDS: Thick, sticky, yellow/green mucus and discharges. Stringy mucus.
Blocked nose.

COUGHS: Croupy, mucusy cough with sticky catarrh which is difficult to
cough up.

HEADACHES AND MIGRAINES: Headaches over eyebrows. Migraines in small
spots.

JOINTS: Joint pains which move across body. Pains occur in small spots.
Sharp stitching pains.

RESPIRATORY ISSUES: Profuse yellow sticky, stringy expectorant which is
very hard to cough up.

SINUSITIS: Sinus headaches with bunged up nose. Pain usually over one eye.

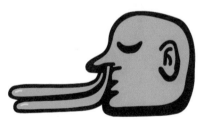

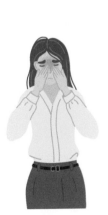

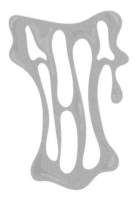

Kali Carb
Childbirth, backaches, respiratory issues

KEY SYMPTOMS:

- Severe backaches before and during period, during pregnancy or labour.
- Back to back labours where labour gets stuck
- Pain feels like back may break
- Swollen, sensitive and painful breasts before period
- Stabbing, stitching pains in chest
- Suffocative choking cough worse at 3am
- Congestive headaches
- Palpitations
- Asthmatic wheezing

backache labours

feels like back will break

stabbing pains

wheezing

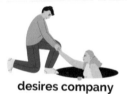

desires company

MENTAL SYMPTOMS

Desires company yet treats them outrageously

Fear of death when alone

Obstinate and dogmatic

EVENT THAT CAUSED SYMPTOMS:

'Never been well since' a cold or pneumonia

Suppression of eruptions in childhood

pneumonia

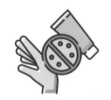

suppressed eruptions

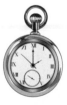

< 2-4am

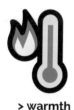

> warmth

Hindered by:
Cold air
2-4am
Lying on painful side
After childbirth

Helped by:
Warm weather
Warmth
Sitting with elbows on knees

Kali Carb
Cheat sheet

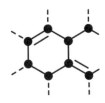
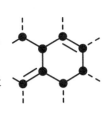

Full name: Kali Carbonicum
Other names: Potassium carbonate, Salt of tartar
Made from the compound potassium carbonate, a white, odourless powder that is soluble in water. In its original form, it is an alkaline substance and has various industrial and chemical applications.

USEFUL FOR:

BACKACHE: As if back is broken. Backache before and during menses. Lower back feels weak. Helped by lying down.

CHILDBIRTH: Useful in backache labours - pain may be felt in back, bum and thighs. Back to back labours where labour gets stuck. Can feel so intense as if back may break. Desires company yet irritable. Helped by firm pressure and warmth.

COUGHS: Dry, hard, choking cough. Worse at 3am. Sharp pains.

RESPIRATORY ISSUES: Shortness of breath especially at night. Wheezing. Helped by sitting up or bending forward. Susceptible to colds. Better in warm climates. Never been well since pneumonia.

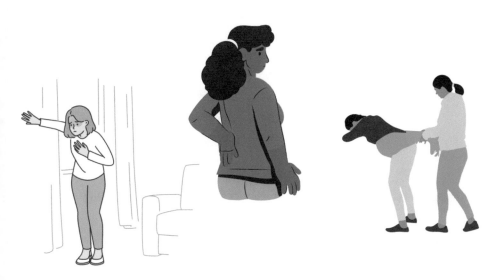

Kali Phos
Exhaustion, overstudy, anxiety

KEY SYMPTOMS:

- Mental and physical weakness caused by overworking
- Slightest task seems like a great effort
- Night terrors
- Excessive blushing
- Sensitive hearing -doesn't like noise
- Humming and buzzing in ears
- Headaches from overstudy
- Cough with yellow phlegm
- Dry mouth
- Diarrhoea caused by fright
- Insomnia from worry

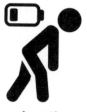

exhaustion

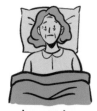

insomnia

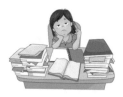

headaches from studying

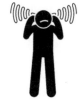

buzzing in ears

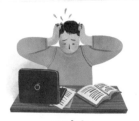

anxiety

MENTAL SYMPTOMS
Anxiety with nervous dread
Brain fatigue

EVENT THAT CAUSED SYMPTOMS:
Overwork
Injuries

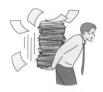

overwork

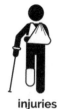

injuries

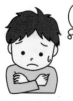

< mental exertion

> warmth

Hindered by:
Mental exertion
Physical exertion
Cold
Puberty
Excitement

Helped by:
Warmth
Rest
Eating

HELP!

Kali Phos
Cheat sheet

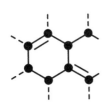

Full name: Kali Phosphoricum
Other names: Potassium phosphate
Made from the chemical compound potassium phosphate. Kali phos is also available as a 'tissue salt' which, although made in line with homeopathic principles (albeit to a less diluted level), still contains a material dose so works on a more physical level. The homeopathic remedy can work on a physical and mental level.

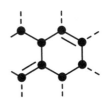

USEFUL FOR:

ANXIETY: Anxiety with a sense of dread. Nervousness. Worried about the future. Fears being alone. May have diarrhoea caused by fright.

EXHAUSTION: Overwork. Mental exhaustion. Brain fatigue.

HEADACHES: Headache due to overstudy. Extreme sensitivity to noise. Pains around the back of head. Helped by gentle motion. Headaches that are worse before menses.

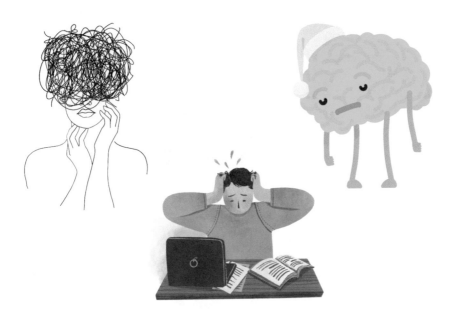

Lachesis
Hot flushes, PMS, sore throats, boils

KEY SYMPTOMS:
- Hemorrhagic tendency
- Flushes of heat
- High blood pressure
- Septic states
- Mottled skin
- Purple membranes
- Sensation of constriction - can't bear tight clothing
- Left sided
- Earache with sore throat
- Sore throat, worse left side and swallowing liquids
- Pre-menstrual symptoms (PMS)

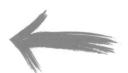

left sided

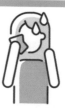

hot flushes

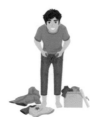

can't stand tight clothing

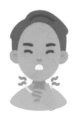

sore throat worse for swallowing

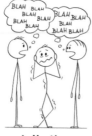

talkative

MENTAL SYMPTOMS
Very talkative
Suspicious
Jealous
Fear of snakes and being poisoned

EVENT THAT CAUSED SYMPTOMS:
Suppressed discharges
Night watching
Loss of fluids
Grief
Jealousy
Menopause

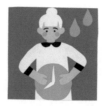

menopause

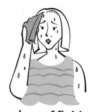

loss of fluids

< swallowing

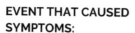

> appearances of discharges

Hindered by:
Swallowing
Hot drinks
After sleep
Suppressed discharges
Morning
Pressure of clothes

Helped by:
Appearance of discharges
Open air
Cold drinks
Loosening clothes
Belching
Eating fruit

Lachesis
Cheat sheet

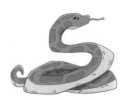

Full name: Lachesis Muta
Other names: Bushmaster snake,
Surukuku
Made from the venom of the
bushmaster snake, a venomous pit
viper found in South America.

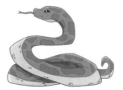

USEFUL FOR:
FEMALE: Premenstrual syndrome. Symptoms go as soon as flow starts.
Cramps and pain which eases when period starts. Violent pain in left ovary.
Flooding periods. Menopause - palpitations. Hot flashes and burning on top
of head. Feels faint. Prolapsed uterus during menopause.

HEADACHES AND MIGRAINES: Headaches before period or during
menopause. Congestive headaches, rush of blood to head.

THROAT: Left sided. Very painful and sore. Pain may extend to ears.
Hindered by touch or pressure. Worse for swallowing saliva or liquid. Pain
worse for hot drinks. Collar and neckband must be loose.

RESPIRATORY ISSUES: Sensation of being strangled. Cannot stand anything
around the neck. Breathing seems to stop when falling asleep.

SKIN: Bluish, purple skin. Boils. Blue-black swellings.

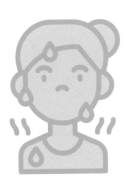

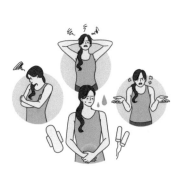

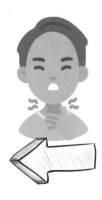

Ledum
Puncture wounds, bites, stings

KEY SYMPTOMS:
- Puncture wounds
- Deep wounds e.g. those caused by nails
- Animal and tick bites
- Numbness or coldness around site
- Swollen, puffy, mottled skin
- Blue and cold-yet feels HOT to the sufferer
- Tearing and throbbing pains
- Gouty pains
- Pains in feet, ankles and soles
- Ankles that sprain easily

puncture wounds

tick bites

blue skin

gouty pains

confusion as if intoxicated

MENTAL SYMPTOMS
Confusion, as if intoxicated
Aversion to friends

EVENT THAT CAUSED SYMPTOMS:
Bites
Puncture wounds

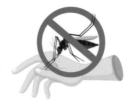

bites

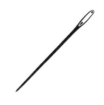

puncture wounds

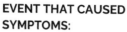

Hindered by:
Warmth

Helped by:
Cold applications

< warmth   **> cold applications**

Ledum
Cheat sheet

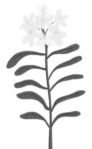

Full name: Ledum Palustre
Other names: Wild rosemary, Marsh tea

This is an evergreen shrub that can be found growing in Europe, Canada and North America. The leaves look similar to the herb rosemary and it flowers in from April to July. The flowers taste bitter and smell of antiseptic.

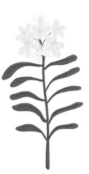

USEFUL FOR:

BITES: Relieves redness, swelling, stinging. Calms the itch of a bite. Prevents septic state setting in.

GOUT: especially of knees and feet. Helped by the cold. Feels hot to the sufferer.

LYME DISEASE: Reputed anti-Lyme properties. If find a tick with head buried, ALWAYS twist and remove, never pull out as it can leave head in and take Ledum 30c.

RHEUMATIC PAINS: Worse from being overheated in bed. Pain and stiffness which is better for cold.

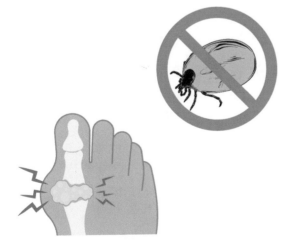

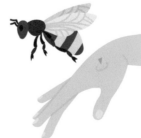

Lycopodium
Bloating, painful periods, liver, low self esteem

KEY SYMPTOMS:

- Bloating and flatulence
- Fermentation in intestines
- Colic in babies
- Eye inflammation
- Painful menses - may faint
- Depression before menses
- Right sided headaches
- Post partum hair loss
- Sciatica, worse right side
- Gallstone colic
- Weak liver
- Craves sweets
- Stools begin hard or constipated then turn soft
- Yellow discharges
- Reverses letters and words

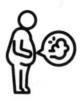
bloating & flatulence

painful menses

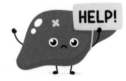 HELP!

sciatica

weak liver

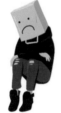

loss of self confidence

MENTAL SYMPTOMS
Low confidence and self esteem
Anxiety - fear of failure
Panic attacks
Domineering to those with less authority

EVENT THAT CAUSED SYMPTOMS:
Domineering parents or siblings
Abuse, fright or mortification
Sugar

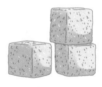
sugar

abuse

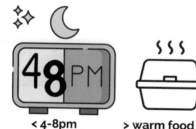

48 PM

< 4-8pm

> warm food

Hindered by:
Right side
Warm room
Pressure of clothes
Oysters, cabbage, beans
4-8pm

Helped by:
Motion
Warm food
Warm drinks

Lycopodium
Cheat sheet

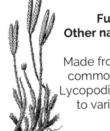

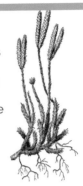

Full name: Lycopodium Clavatum
Other names: Club moss, Wolf's claw, Muscus terrestris repens
Made from the spores of the plant Lycopodium commonly known as club moss or wolf's foot. Lycopodium is a small, creeping plant. It is native to various regions, including Europe, North America and parts of Asia.

USEFUL FOR:

EARS: Itching in ear. Thick yellow discharges.

EYES: Eyes feel too large. Photophobia. Eye inflammation. Painful, bruised sensation. Styes on lids.

FEMALE: Painful periods with fainting. Pains in right ovary or from right to left. Clotty dark menses.

LIVER: Jaundice with flatulence. Weak liver and poor digestion. Violent gallstone colic.

STOMACH: Weakness of digestion. Gas and bloating. Worse 4-8pm. Acidic belchings. Fermentation in intestines. Craves sweets but all symptoms worse for them. Constipation. Colic in babies. Noisy flatulence. Hypoglycemia. Allergies to wheat.

THROAT: Sore throat which is helped by warm drinks. Hindered by cold drinks. Right sided or moves from right to left. Throat feels cold. Sensation as if a ball rose up in throat. Ulceration of tonsils.

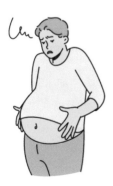

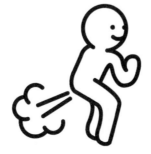

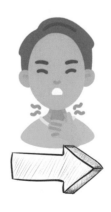

Mag Phos
Cramps, pain

KEY SYMPTOMS:

- Cramps and neuralgic pain
- Period pains helped by a hot water bottle
- Colic in babies
- Wind and excess gas
- Face neuralgia (shooting, stabbing)
- Better bending double
- Writer's cramp
- Twitching - eyes or legs
- Sciatica
- Cramping of muscles with radiating pains
- Growing pains
- Teething

cramps

wind & gas

period pains

colic

oversensitive

MENTAL SYMPTOMS

Oversensitive to pain, noise or excitement
Anxiety from the pains

EVENT THAT CAUSED SYMPTOMS:

Teething
Overuse of muscles

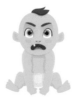

teething

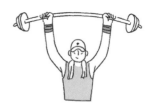

overexertion

< cold air

> heat

Hindered by:
Cold air
Uncovering
Night
Touch

Helped by:
Heat
Warmth
Pressure
Bending double
Standing up

Mag Phos
Cheat sheet

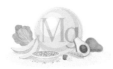

Full name: Magnesium Phosphorica
Other names: Magnesium phosphate
Made from the mineral compound Magnesium phosphate, a naturally occurring mineral that is present in various body tissues.
Mag phos is also available as a 'tissue salt' which, although made in line with homeopathic principles (albeit to a less diluted level), still contains a material dose so works on a more physical level. The homeopathic remedy can work on a physical and mental level.

USEFUL FOR:

FACIAL NEURALGIA: Right sided. Helped by heat and pressure.

PERIOD PAINS: Helped by a hot water bottle and rubbing.

SPASMS AND ANY CRAMPS: Such as stomach cramps, eye twitching, writer's cramp or leg cramps.

STOMACH ISSUES: Wind helped by rubbing and warmth but not by belching. Colic in babies.

TOOTHACHE: Helped by hot drinks.

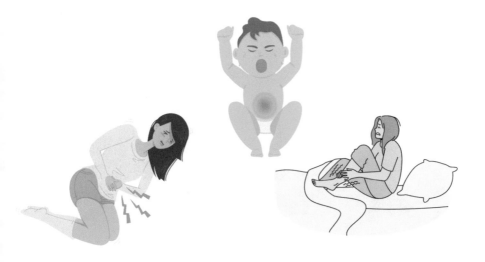

Merc
Sore throats, ear infections, mouth ulcers

KEY SYMPTOMS:
- Human thermometers - sensitive to both heat and cold
- Enlarged lymphatic glands
- Ulcerations of mouth and throat
- Sore throat - pain on swallowing
- Quinsy - abscess on tonsil
- Foul discharges which may be green or blood streaked
- Excessive saliva
- Ear pain that extends to teeth
- Swimmers or glue ear
- Thirsty for cold drinks
- Catarrhal headaches - as if bandaged
- Metallic taste in mouth

ulcers

human thermometers

excessive saliva

foul discharges

irresolute

MENTAL SYMPTOMS
Changes mind constantly
Restlessness especially at night

EVENT THAT CAUSED SYMPTOMS:
Fright
Suppressed sweat

fright

suppressed sweat

< night

> moderate climate

Hindered by:
Drafts
Taking cold
Damp weather
Night
Right side
Heat
Changing weather

Helped by:
Moderate temperature

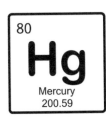

Merc
Cheat sheet

80
Hg
Mercury
200.59

Full name: Mercurius Solublis
Other names: Mercury vivus,
Mercury solublis, Quicksilver,
Argentum vivum
Made from the chemical element
Mercury, a heavy, silver-white metal
that is liquid at room temperature.

80
Hg
Mercury
200.59

USEFUL FOR:
BOILS AND ABSCESSES: Offensive eruptions.

CHICKEN POX: Worse from the warmth of bed. Itchy. Easily bleeding.

COLD SORES, CANKER SORES: Bloody discharges. Bad breath. Excessive
saliva. Thirsty.

CONJUNCTIVITIS: From taking cold. Burning or acrid discharge.

EAR INFECTIONS: acute and chronic. Swimmers ear or glue ear. Pain may
radiate from throat to ears. Discharges may be streaked with blood.
Thirsty, Sensitive to heat and cold. Worse at night. Sweaty.

GUM DISORDERS: Gingivitis.

SINUSITIS: Catarrhal headaches. Burning and pulsations in forehead.

SORE THROATS: Foul breath, pain on swallowing, pain extends to ears.
Enlarged glands. Throat raw, dry, burning or stinging. Increased salivation.
Tongue imprinted with teeth. Metallic taste in mouth.

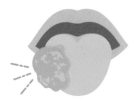

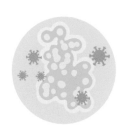

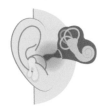

Mixed pollens
Hayfever

KEY SYMPTOMS:
- Can help with hayfever symptoms
- Any reactions to pollens
- Tree, grass and flower allergies
- Watery eyes
- Runny nose
- Stinging
- Burning
- Sneezing

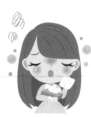

hayfever

any reactions to pollens

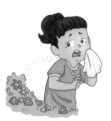

sneezing or runny nose

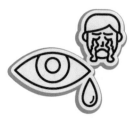

watery eyes

Mixed pollens
Hayfever

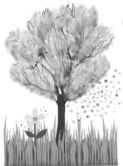

Mixed pollens is a homeopathic remedy made from a mixture of pollens from trees, grasses and flowers.

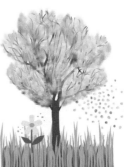

Mixed pollens tends to be prescribed therapeutically so accompanying symptoms, event that caused complaint and helped or hindered are not generally taken into account when deciding whether to give this remedy.

DOSING

Take during hayfever season. Follow regular homeopathic dosing principles. If frequent dosing is needed then add one pellet to a bottle of water - one sip equals one dose (and this one sip is equivalent to one pill). Can be used in the morning as a preventative.

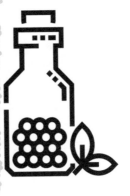

Natrum Mur
Cold sores, mouth ulcers, colds, headaches

- **KEY SYMPTOMS:**
- Streaming colds with sneezing and discharge from the eyes
- Loss of taste or smell
- Cold sores
- Mouth ulcers
- Headaches and migraines 'like hammers beating the head'
- Dry lips - cracks in the corners
- Watering eyes worse in wind
- Colitis with sudden urging
- Bleeding haemorrhoids
- Craves salt
- Aggravation from the sun
- 'Bashful kidneys' unable to urinate in front of others
- Back pain helped by lying on something hard

cold sores & mouth ulcers

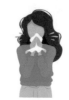

headache 'like hammers beating the head'

craves salt

streaming colds with sneezing

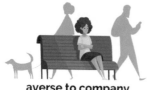

averse to company

MENTAL SYMPTOMS
Closed and affected by grief
Sad yet unable to weep or involuntary weeping
Aversion to company

EVENT THAT CAUSED SYMPTOMS:
Grief
Guilt
Betrayal or disappointment
Sunlight

grief

sunlight

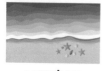

< seashore

> fasting

Hindered by:
Sunlight
Seashore
9-11am
Music

Helped by:
Sweating
Going without regular meals

Natrum Mur
Cheat sheet

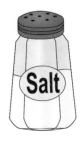

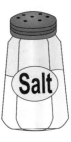

Full name: Natrum Muriaticum
Other names: Sodium chloride,
table or common rock salt
Made from the naturally occurring mineral compound Sodium chloride. It is widely distributed in nature, and its primary source for homeopathic preparations is usually sea salt or rock salt.

USEFUL FOR:

BACK PAIN: Desire for firm support. Bruising pain. Spine oversensitive to touch.

COLD SORES, CANKER SORES: May have dry or cracked lips. Worse for sunlight.

COLDS: Streaming colds with discharge from eyes and lots of sneezing. Thickens up after a few days and then feels stuffed up and unable to taste or smell.

GRIEF: Acute and chronic. Emotionally shut down.

HAYFEVER: Streaming, bland discharge from eyes and nose. Sneezing. Loss of taste or smell. Irritated by the sun.

HEADACHES AND MIGRAINES: Like hammers hitting the head. May crave salt. Worse for company, light, sun, noise and reading. Worse at 10am. Headache from grief. Helped by lying in a dark room, cold applications and sweating. Numbness in face or lips before headache. Visual disturbances before headache.

STOMACH: Anxiety in abdomen. Weakness in the stomach, comes in spells. Morning sickness with vomiting, watery, frothy phlegm. Hard, difficult and painful stool followed by liquid stool. Dry, hard or crumbling stool. Irregular stools.

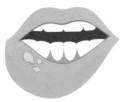

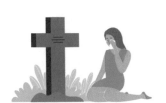

Nux Vomica
Hangover, indigestion, irritability

KEY SYMPTOMS:

- Heartburn
- Hangovers
- Nausea with lots of retching
- Heavy stomach - sensitive to touch
- Wind and bloating
- Constipation due to reverse peristaltic action
- Morning diarrhoea after a heavy binge
- Migraines where brain feels bruised
- Liver issues
- Colds - stuffy nose at night, runny in day
- Flu with backache, shivering and sweating
- Insomnia - worrying about work
- Waking 3-4am

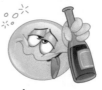

hangover

nausea
(but can't bring
anything up)

colds that are
free flowing
inside but stuffed
up outside

heavy stomach
after eating,
bloated

irritable

MENTAL SYMPTOMS
Ambitious workaholic
Headstrong
Irritable and angry
Sensitivity- noise, odours, light, music

**EVENT THAT CAUSED
SYMPTOMS:**
Alcohol
Drugs
Spices
Sexual excess

alcohol

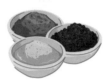

spices

< noise

> night

Hindered by:
Morning
Cold air
Noise
Overeating

Helped by:
Heat
Evening
Rest
Damp weather

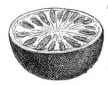 # Nux Vomica
Cheat sheet

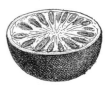

Other names: Poison Nut, Strychnos nux vomica

Made from Strychnos nux vomica, a deciduous tree native to India and to South East Asia. It is a medium-sized tree in the family Loganiaceae that grows in open habitats. The seeds contain strychnine and are extremely bitter.

USEFUL FOR:

BLADDER: Cystitis with constant urging, helped by warmth and warm baths. Relieved for moments only on passing small quantities of urine.

COLDS: Sneezing and runny nose on waking. Blocked up nose outside, free flowing inside.

FLU: High fever and violent chills. Worse from movement. Very sensitive to drafts.

HANGOVERS: all hangover symptoms which may include headache and nausea.

HAY FEVER: Lots of sneezing, streaming from eyes and nose. Irritable. Hindered by dry air and helped by a damp atmosphere.

HEADACHES AND MIGRAINE: Worse for noise, light and mental effort. Worse before period. Photophobia.

INSOMNIA: Wakes around 3-4am and cannot sleep due to thoughts about work. Sleepiness during the day.

PERIOD PAINS: Pain in sacrum and constant urging for stools. Cramping causing to double up and cry. Must stay in bed. Uterine spasms with discharge of clots.

STOMACH: Nausea but can't bring anything up. Bloating for hours after eating. Heavy stomach. Loves rich and fatty foods and tolerates it well. May have stomach ulcers. Morning diarrhoea after a heavy binge. Constipation due to reverse action of the gut rather than stool being too large or dry.

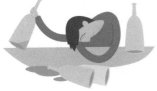 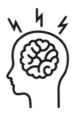

Opium
Shock, ailments without pain, constipation

KEY SYMPTOMS:
- Lack of reaction
- Loss of consciousness
- Retained or involuntary urination after a fright
- Fixed pupils that don't react to light
- Hot face
- Deep rattling snoring
- Constipation with round, black, hard balls
- Twitching of limbs
- Drowsiness
- PTSD remedy - may be jumpy
- Insomnia where they wake at every noise yet very sleepy in the day

PTSD

constipation where history of trauma

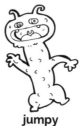

jumpy

insomnia

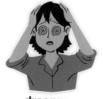

dreamy

MENTAL SYMPTOMS
Dreamy, detached and dull feelings
Confusion
Unable to appreciate her suffering
Nervous, irritable or jumpy

EVENT THAT CAUSED SYMPTOMS:
Fright
Shame
Drug overdose

fright   **shame**

< suppressed discharges

> cold

Hindered by:
Suppressed discharges
Alcohol
After sleep

Helped by:
Cold
Uncovering
Constant walking

Opium
Cheat sheet

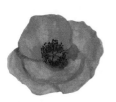

Other names: Poppy, Papaver officinale
Made from the opium poppy, a flowering plant that is well-known for producing opium, a natural substance that contains various alkaloids, including morphine and codeine.

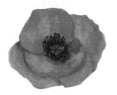

USEFUL FOR:

CONSTIPATION: Round, hard stools like black balls. Bloody mucus. Desire to pass stool absent. Unfinished feeling. Constipation in babies where there has been a traumatic birth.

KIDNEYS: Retained or involuntary urination after a fright.

PAIN: Any ailments without pain.

PTSD: especially useful in cases of post-natal depression if there has been a traumatic birth. Dreamy, detached and dull feelings. Drowsiness or confusion. Unable to appreciate her suffering. Nervous, irritable or jumpy.

INSOMNIA: Wakes at every noise yet very sleepy in the day.

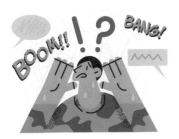

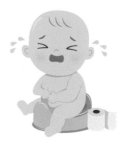

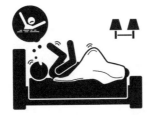

Phos Ac
Grief, diarrhoea, fatigue, hair loss, homesickness

KEY SYMPTOMS:
- Loss of vital fluids (sweat, urine, diarrhoea)
- Weakness and debility
- Weak feeling in chest from talking
- Blue rings around the eyes
- Pain as if eyeballs were forcibly pressed together into head
- Frequent urination at night
- Profuse painless watery stools
- Hair loss, especially after grief
- Sweaty
- Vertigo towards the evening
- Craves Cola drinks

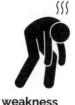
weakness

loss of vital fluids

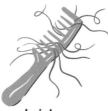
hair loss

blue rings around eyes

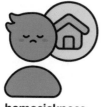
homesickness

MENTAL SYMPTOMS
Grief - overwhelmed by grief
Homesickness

EVENT THAT CAUSED SYMPTOMS:
Bad news
Grief
Sexual excess
Loss of fluids

loss of fluids

grief

< loss of vital fluids

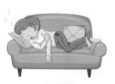
> nap

Hindered by:
Loss of vital fluids
Cold drafts
Music
Being away from home

Helped by:
Warmth
After short sleep
After passing stool

Phos Ac
Cheat sheet

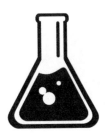
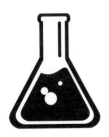

Full name: Phosphoricum Acidum
Made from the chemical compound Phosphoric acid, a mineral acid that is derived from phosphorus, a non-metallic element. It is a weak acid and is commonly found in various foods and beverages, including soft drinks. In its concentrated form, it is corrosive and can be harmful.

USEFUL FOR:

DIARRHOEA: Profuse thin watery stools. Painless stools. White stools. Involuntary stools.

EXHAUSTION: Nervous exhaustion. Debility. Slowness of mind. Impaired memory. Can't find the right words. Indifferent to everything. Aversion to talking. Wants to be left alone.

GRIEF: Silent grief. Wants to be alone. Aversion to loved ones. Apathetic.

HAIR LOSS: Especially if after a grief.

HOMESICKNESS: Longs for home. Insomnia and pining.

INSOMNIA: Sleep by day. Awake at night.

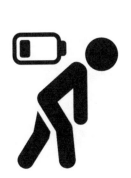
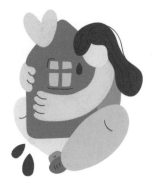
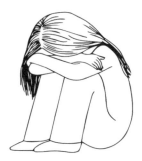

Phosphorus
Vomiting, diarrhoea, bleeding, anxiety

KEY SYMPTOMS:

- Hemorrhagic tendency
- Nosebleeds
- Exhausting diarrhoea
- Vomiting - water thrown up as soon as it hits the stomach
- Debility and collapse states
- Easily dehydrated with tremendous thirst
- Chemical sensitivity
- Craves ice cream or cold drinks
- Ravenous hunger during fever
- Hoarseness usually without pain
- Respiratory infections - every cold goes to chest
- Tightness in chest
- Tickly cough
- Numbness of fingers

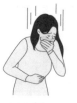

vomiting

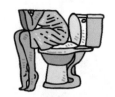

exhausting diarrhoea

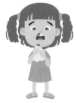

nosebleeds

thirsty for icy cold drinks

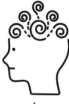

anxious

MENTAL SYMPTOMS
Anxiety
Open and suggestible
Fearful of being alone, dark, death, thunderstorms
Health anxiety (easily reassured)

EVENT THAT CAUSED SYMPTOMS:
Grief
Rain
Iodine
Electrocution

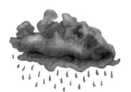

rain

grief

< fasting

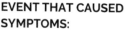

> eating

Hindered by:
Fasting
Lying on left side
Spicy foods,
Salt
Thunderstorms
Mental exertion
Loss of fluids

Helped by:
Eating
Cold drinks
Sleep
Sympathy

Phosphorus
Cheat sheet

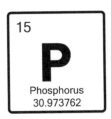

15

P

Phosphorus
30.973762

Other names: White phosphorus
Phosphorus is a non-metallic element and is found in various forms in nature. It is essential for life and is present in the cells of living organisms. In its elemental form, phosphorus is highly reactive and can spontaneously ignite in air, which is why it is typically stored under water or in an inert atmosphere.

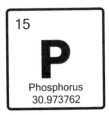

15

P

Phosphorus
30.973762

USEFUL FOR:

ANXIETY: Sensitive, Suggestible. Wants company. Fear of darkness, death and thunderstorms. Health anxiety.

COUGHS AND RESPIRATORY ISSUES: Pneumonia. Worse lying on left side. Rusty coloured sputum. Body trembles. Quickened breathing. Feels as if a weight on chest. Tightness across chest. heat in the chest. Lingering, tickling coughs.

DIARRHOEA: Exhausting diarrhoea. Great weakness after stools. Stools difficult to expel. May be blood streaked, watery and profuse.

EXHAUSTION: Wants sympathy. Nervous exhaustion. Spacey.

FEVER: Ravenous hunger during fever. Craving for ice cold drinks or ice cream.

HEADACHES: Headaches with sensitivity to smells. Hunger before or during headache. Coldness of occiput. Heat comes up from spine. Strained feeling of eyes.

NOSEBLEEDS: Number 1 remedy for nosebleeds.

THROAT: Tendency to get sore throats that go to the chest. Lost voice in singers. Rawness and scraping in throat. Tickling in larynx. Sweet taste when coughing.

VOMITING: Post op vomiting. Water thrown up as soon as it hits the stomach.

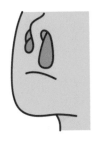
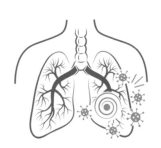
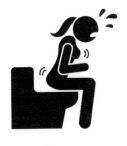

Phytolacca
Number 1 for breast issues, glands, sore throats

KEY SYMPTOMS:
- Shooting pains like electric shocks
- Sore, hard, aching pains
- Glandular swellings with heat and inflammation
- Number 1 remedy for cracked nipples, blocked milk ducts and mastitis
- Hot, full and tender breasts - armpit glands may be swollen
- Mastitis with flu like symptoms - pale and shivery
- Rheumatism after tonsillitis
- Right sided sore throats

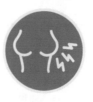

Number 1 for breast issues

mastitis with flu symptoms

shooting pains

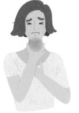

right sided sore throats

restless

MENTAL SYMPTOMS
Irritable and nervous
Restless
Melancholy

EVENT THAT CAUSED SYMPTOMS:
Grief
Injuries
Exposure to cold, damp weather

damp weather

grief

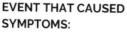

< **swallowing**

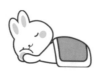

> **lying on tummy**

Hindered by:
Damp cold weather
Rain
Movement
Swallowing

Helped by:
Warmth
Dry weather
Lying on abdomen

Phytolacca
Cheat sheet

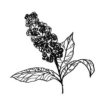
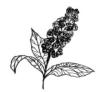

HELP!

Full name: Phytolacca Decandra
Other names: Poke root, Poke weed, Virginian poke, Pole-root, Garget weed, Red ink plant
The homeopathic remedy Phytolacca is made from the plant Phytolacca decandra, commonly known as poke root. Phytolacca is a perennial plant native to North America, South America and East Asia.

USEFUL FOR:

BREAST ISSUES: Number 1 remedy for cracked nipples, blocked milk ducts and mastitis. Intense pains that radiate out from nipple sometimes into arm. Hot, full and tender breasts. Armpit glands may be swollen. Breasts swollen and heavy. Flu like symptoms - pale and shivery. May have blood in milk. Helped by breast feeding.

JOINT PAINS: Pains like electric shocks. Wandering pains. Pains come and go. Muscle soreness.

THROAT: Raw, sore throat. Swollen tonsils. Throat feels rough, narrow and hot. Shooting pains into ears on swallowing. Cannot swallow anything hot. Painful on swallowing. Sensation of hot ball or lump. Quinsy. Worse right side.

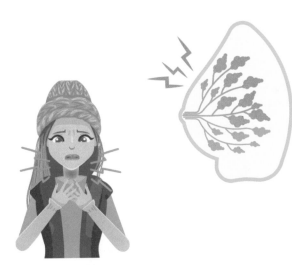
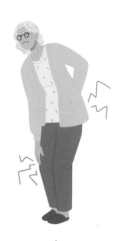

Pulsatilla
Queen of Remedies, changeable, catarrh, clinginess

KEY SYMPTOMS:
- Changing, shifting symptoms
- One sided problems
- Mucus membranes
- Thick, bland, green or yellow discharges
- Thirstless
- Dry mouth and lips
- Chilly yet intolerant of heat
- Desires fresh air
- Never been well since puberty
- Bandaged sensation or as if part were growing too large
- Hormonal issues including morning sickness
- Teething where child is clingy

changeable symptoms

fevers where mouth & lips are dry

thick green or yellow catarrh

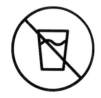

No thirst

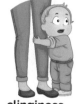

clinginess

MENTAL SYMPTOMS
Yielding like the windflower
Weepy and tearful
Desires sympathy
Clinginess

EVENT THAT CAUSED SYMPTOMS:
Getting feet wet
Abandonment
Rich or fatty foods such as ice cream, pork, fats, pastry
Suppressed menses

getting feet wet

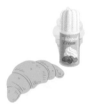

fatty foods

< stuffy rooms

> fresh air

Hindered by:
Rich food
Puberty
Before menses
Pregnancy
Twilight
Sunset
Stuffy rooms

Helped by:
Fresh air
Crying
Gentle motion
Cold compress
Sympathy
Attention

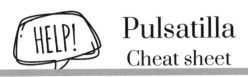
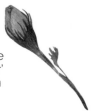

Pulsatilla
Cheat sheet

Full name: Pulsatilla Nigrans
Other names: Wind flower, Pasque flower,
Anenome pratensis

Pulsatilla is also known as the Pasque flower because
it blooms around Easter times (pasque means 'Easter'
in French). It grows in Europe, prefers chalky calcium
rich soil and is found in open situations.

USEFUL FOR:

CHICKEN POX: especially when weepy and clingy.

COUGHS, COLDS AND UPPER RESPIRATORY INFECTIONS: accompanied by thick
green or yellow discharges often from one nostril. Needs attention. May have
started after getting feet wet. A dry cough at night and a loose cough in the
morning. Thirstless. Changeable symptoms.

CYSTITIS: bladder pain, worse at the end of urination or if trying to retain urine.

EAR INFECTIONS: Number 1 remedy for childhood ear infections. Tearful and
clingy. Pain is worse at night. Diminished hearing. Pulsating pain. Discharges from
the ear. Needs consolation.

EYES: Conjunctivitis or styes. May have greenish discharge from eyes. Itching and
pain in eye. Helped by cold applications.

FEMALE: Hot flushes. Piles during menopause. Painful but scanty periods. PMS and
painful breasts. Nausea. Morning sickness. Weepy and desires company.

FEVERS: where mouths and lips are dry but thirstless. Chilly yet intolerant of heat.

HAYFEVER: Thick, bland discharges. May have one side of nose blocked.

HEADACHES AND MIGRAINES: May appear during the end of period. Vertigo.
Hindered by looking upwards, stuffy rooms. Helped by lying down, cold, open air.

SINUSITIS: As if a nail is driven in. Desire to press the head against something.

STOMACH: Indigestion from fats and rich foods. Thirstless.

TEETHING: Weepy and clingy. Unable to sleep wants company.

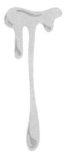
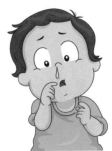

Rhus Tox
The 'Swiss Army Knife', sprains, rashes, chicken pox

KEY SYMPTOMS:
- Number 1 for chicken pox
- Hindered by first movement, helped by continued motion - **like a 'rusty gate'**
- Stiffness with restlessness
- Joint pains - bruised and sore
- Tearing and shooting pains
- Swollen joints from overexertion
- Restlessness - can't get comfy in any position
- Flu where can't get comfy
- Thirsty for cold milk or water which may be vomited
- Rheumatic pains especially in cold damp season
- Skin irritations especially of the face, scalp, genitals and mucus membranes
- Cold sores

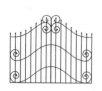

< first movement
> continued motion
like a rusty gate

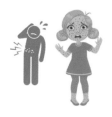

shingles & chicken pox

stiffness

tearing & shooting pains

superstitious

MENTAL SYMPTOMS
Superstitious
Restlessness
Weeping, without knowing why
Apprehension at night

EVENT THAT CAUSED SYMPTOMS:
Strains
Over lifting
Getting wet
Cold bathing
Change of weather to cold or damp

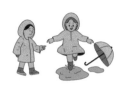

getting wet

strains

< first movement   **> continued motion**

Hindered by:
First movement
Cold
Damp
Before storms
Change of weather

Helped by:
Continued motion
Stretching
Rubbing or holding affected part
Heat and warmth

HELP!

Rhus Tox
Cheat sheet

Full name: Rhus Toxicodendron
Other names: Poison oak, Poison ivy,
Toxicodendron radicans
The homeopathic remedy Rhus tox is made from the plant Toxicodendron radicans, commonly known as poison ivy. Poison ivy is a woody vine or shrub predominantly found in North America.

USEFUL FOR:

CHICKEN POX / SHINGLES: first choice remedy for chicken pox or shingles.

COLD SORES: of mouth or genitals. Blisters around lips.

EYES: Orbital cellulitis. Hot scalding tears. Yellow pus. Photophobia. Styes on lower lids.

FLU: Restlessness, aches and pains. Helped by warmth and continued motion.

PAINS/STRAINS/SPRAINS: Restless legs. Sciatica. Helped by hot baths, continued motion. All pains worse on the first movement. Hindered by damp weather. Cracking joints.

SKIN ISSUES: Itching is helped by scalding hot water. Useful for herpes and shingles. First choice for poison ivy rash. Urticaria.

STREP INFECTIONS: Has 'anti-strep' properties so useful for Scarlet Fever and sore throats.

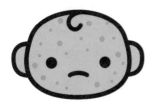

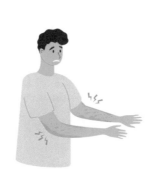

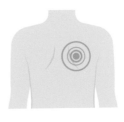

Ruta
Sprains, strains, bruised bones

KEY SYMPTOMS:
- Deep aching pain
- Bruises to the lining of bones
- Remedy for overuse - eyestrain/prolapse
- Deeper acting than Rhus Tox but with a less distinctive picture (less restless)
- Sore and aching, bones as if broken
- Bruised sensation
- Injured joints especially bruised bones
- Torn and wrenched tendons
- Lameness after sprains
- Loss of elasticity in muscles and tendons

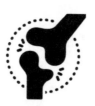

bruising to lining of bones

bruised sensation

injured joints

torn tendons

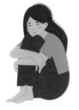

despair

MENTAL SYMPTOMS
Weakness
Despair

EVENT THAT CAUSED SYMPTOMS:
Carrying heavy weights
Overuse of tendons
Going up and downstairs

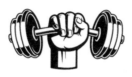

heavy weights

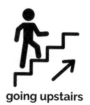

going upstairs

< eyestrain

> gentle movement

Hindered by:
Overexertion
Eyestrain

Helped by:
Warmth
Gentle movement

Ruta
Cheat sheet

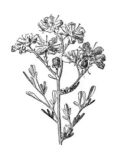

Full name: Ruta Graveolens
Other names: Garden rue, Bitterwort
Ruta graveolens is a perennial herb with a long history of medicinal use and is native to Southern Europe. The plant has bluish-green leaves and produces small, yellow flowers.

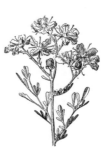

USEFUL FOR:

EYESTRAIN: Dim weak eyesight. Strained and aching eyes. May have a headache due to eyestrain.

PAINS/STRAINS/SPRAINS: Injured joints. Torn tendons. Bruised bones. Sore. Aching with restlessness. Heaviness. Overexertion. Helped by lying on back. Slipped vertebrae. Hamstrings feel shortened. Knees give way. Ganglion wrist.

PROLAPSES: Prolapsed uterus. Rectal prolapse.

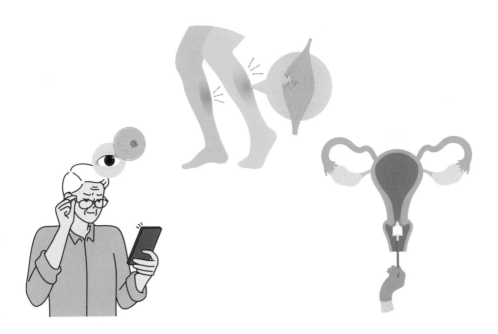

Sabadilla
Hayfever

KEY SYMPTOMS:
- One of the top hayfever remedies where both EYES and NOSE are affected
- Acts on mucus membranes especially of nose and eyes
- Red eyes
- Burning eyes
- Spasmodic sneezing with running nose
- Copious watery discharges
- Chilliness
- Sensitive to cold
- Sore throat which starts on left side
- Periodicity
- Thirstless
- Desires hot things
- Pinworms

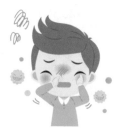

hayfever

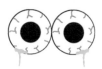

red eyes

runny nose

chilliness

nervous

MENTAL SYMPTOMS
Nervous
Timid
Easily startled
Hypochrondria

EVENT THAT CAUSED SYMPTOMS:
Fright
Overthinking
Pinworms

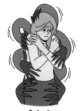

fright

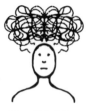

overthinking

< cold

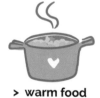

> warm food

Hindered by:
Cold
Cold drinks
Full moon

Helped by:
Warm food
Warm drinks
Being wrapped up

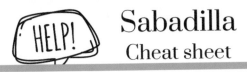

Sabadilla
Cheat sheet

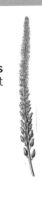

Full name: Sabadilla Officinalis
Other names: Cevadilla seed, Cebadilla,
Asagrae officinalis. Schoenocaulon officinalis
Made from the Cevadilla, a flowering plant that
belongs to the Melanthiaceae family. It is a
perennial plant native to Mexico and Central
America.

USEFUL FOR:

HAYFEVER: Hay fever, characterized by prominent sneezing. Sore
eyes and nose. Red burning eyelids. Persistent, abortive, violent, or
spasmodic sneezing during hay fever episodes. The condition may
be triggered by the fragrance of flowers or freshly mown grass.
Sinus issues. Itching, tingling, and tickling sensations are present,
leading to an irresistible urge to rub the affected areas.

RECTUM: Burning stools. Pinworms.

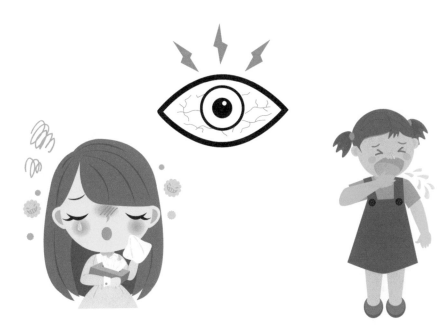

Secale
Childbirth essential, uterus complaints

KEY SYMPTOMS:
- Sensitive to cold but can't bear to be covered
- Hemorrhages
- Weakness
- Burning skin
- Intolerant of stuffy rooms
- Stupefied in labour
- Long contractions
- Threatened miscarriage
- Olive green, thin, bloody stools
- Burning skin with aversion to heat
- Antidotes ill effect of Syntometrine (the drug given routinely to speed up expulsion of placenta)
- Retained placenta
- Gangrene - feels cold

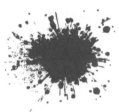

bleeding

retained placenta

intolerant of stuffy rooms

gangrene

suspicious

MENTAL SYMPTOMS
Restless
Anxious
Suspicious

EVENT THAT CAUSED SYMPTOMS:
Miscarriage
Childbirth
Suppression of tears
Wounds

miscarriage

childbirth

< heat

> cold

Hindered by:
Heat
Warmth
Before period
Pregnancy

Helped by:
Cold
Open air
Uncovering

Secale
Cheat sheet

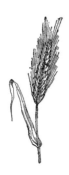 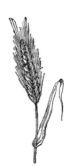

Full name: Secale Cornutum
Other names: Ergot of rye,
Spurred rye, Claviceps purpurea
The homeopathic remedy Secale is made from the fungus Claviceps purpurea, commonly known as ergot. Ergot is a parasitic fungus that affects certain types of grasses, particularly rye.

USESFUL FOR:
CHILDBIRTH: Anxious and restless. Sensitive to cold. Feels weak. Skin may feel like it is burning. Intolerant of stuffy rooms (like Pulsatilla). Stupefied in labour. Long contractions, trembling in between. May lose a little blood with each contraction.

Antidotes ill effect of Syntometrine (the drug given routinely to speed up expulsion of placenta) - take immediately after where possible

Can also be used to encourage a retained placenta to be pushed out naturally.

FEMALE: Continuous oozing of dark, watery blood. Bearing down pains with coldness. Period pains with intolerance of heat.

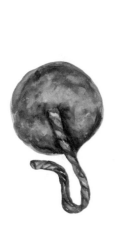 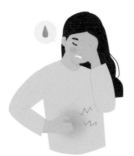 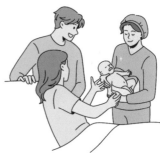

Sepia
Hormonal issues, post natal depression, prolapses

KEY SYMPTOMS:

- Nausea and vomiting in pregnancy
- Hormonal disorders - hot flushes, low libido, menstruation disorders, vaginitis, hair loss at menopause
- Post partum depression
- Prolapses (uterus or bladder) - bearing down sensation
- Weakness in small of back
- Chloasma (yellow saddle across face)
- Aversion to company yet dreads being alone
- Genital warts or herpes
- Restless limbs
- Constipation - shooting pains
- Left sided headaches
- Cracking of lip corners or lower middle lip
- 'Ball' sensation in inner parts

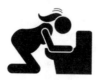

morning sickness

hormonal issues

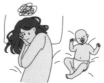

post partum depression

prolapses

worn out

MENTAL SYMPTOMS
Mentally and physically worn out
Tearful or involuntary weeping
Indifferent to family
Irritable and angry

EVENT THAT CAUSED SYMPTOMS:
Overwork
Hormonal changes such as puberty, pregnancy, menopause, contraceptive pill

overwork

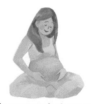

hormonal changes

< before thunderstorms

> exercise

Hindered by:
Cold air
Left side
Before thunderstorms
Before period
Housework

Helped by:
Exercise
Dancing or vigorous motion
Warmth of bed

Sepia
Cheat sheet

Full name: Sepia Succus
Other names: Cuttlefish ink, Sepia officinalis
Sepia is the name given to brown- black ink derived from the cuttlefish. It was used in Hahnemann's time as an artists' pigment and he observed that his sickly artist friend often licked his paintbrush as he worked.

USEFUL FOR:
FEMALE: Irregular menstrual cycles with heavy, painful periods. Flooding. Backache. Bearing down pain in pelvic region. Irritable - aversion to family. Aversion to sex. PMS with irritability, mood swings, and fatigue. Menopause - hot flashes which start in pelvis. Night sweats during menopause. Vaginal dryness and discomfort.

MIND: Feelings of sadness, indifference or apathy towards loved ones. Easily fatigued mentally and physically, with aversion to work and responsibilities. Irritability and anger, especially towards family members. Desire for solitude and aversion to company. Mental exhaustion with difficulty in concentrating or remembering things.

NAUSEA: Faint sinking feeling. Thought of food makes nauseous. Morning sickness.

PROLAPSES: Number 1 remedy for prolapses. Bladder or uterus. Bearing down sensation.

RECTUM: Sensation of ball in anus. Shooting pains up rectum and vagina. Hemorrhoids during pregnancy. Constipation during pregnancy.

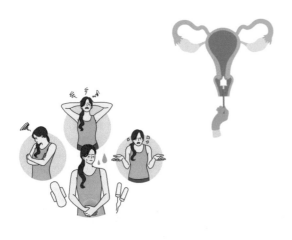

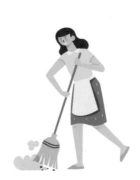

Silica
Splinters, poor assimilation

KEY SYMPTOMS:
- Weakness and fatigue
- Poor assimilation of nutrition leading to defects of bone, skin, hair, nails and teeth
- Sweats on scalp
- Chilly
- 'Bashful stool' which seems to recede after nearly extruding
- Infants unable to tolerate mothers milk
- Abscess formation anywhere
- Enlarged hard glands
- Helps body eliminate
- Tear duct infections
- Sinus headaches
- Acne which leaves small pits in the face
- Hair loss

splinters

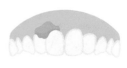

abscesses

aids elimination

sinus headaches

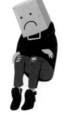

lack of self confidence

MENTAL SYMPTOMS
Yielding, refined, delicate
Lack of self confidence
Conscientiousness
Mental dullness
Fear of needles

EVENT THAT CAUSED SYMPTOMS:
Suppressed sweat
Loss of fluids
Splinters
Overwork

suppressed sweat

splinters

< cold air

> warmth

Hindered by:
Cold air, drafts
Combing hair
Mental exertion
Suppressed sweat
Moon changes

Helped by:
Warmth
Summer
Profuse urination
Magnetism and electricity

Silica
Cheat sheet

Full name: Silica Terra
Other names: Pure flint, Silex,
Silicon dioxide
Made from Silicon dioxide, a compound
commonly found in nature such as
quartz or sand.

USEFUL FOR:

BONES AND JOINTS: Back pain with a sensation of weakness or instability. Joint pains that worsen in cold and damp weather. Weak bones.

CONSTIPATION: Chronic constipation with difficulty passing stool. Gastric disturbances with a feeling of fullness and bloating after eating. 'Bashful stool' which seems to recede after nearly extruding. Sensitivity to milk.

EARS: Pus, glue ear. Itching, tingling, shooting pain. Popping sounds.

GLANDS: Swollen lymph nodes, particularly in the neck and throat area. Glandular infections and inflammations.

HEAD: Headaches located over one eye. Sick headaches. Must keep head covered. or catches a cold. Sweats on head. Hair loss. Premature balding.

MIND: Lack of self-confidence and assertiveness. Easily fatigued, physically and mentally, from exertion. Timidity and shyness in social situations.

SKIN AND NAILS: Slow healing of wounds and skin infections. Nail problems, such as brittle, weak, or deformed nails. Boils, abscesses, or styes that are slow to develop and slow to heal. Splinters - helps remove foreign bodies. Keloid scars.

TEETH: Toothache with sensitivity to cold or touch.

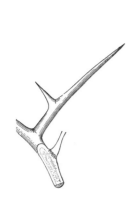 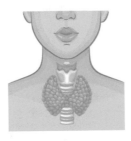 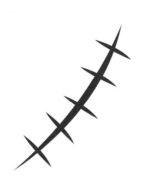

Spongia
Croup, whooping cough, swelling of glands

KEY SYMPTOMS:
- Dry, barking, croupy cough
- Whooping cough
- Suffocative breathing
- Great hunger
- Swelling of glands
- Sensation of heart surging
- Dryness of airways
- Starting from sleep
- Anxiety
- Sensation as if a plug in larynx
- Hoarseness

croup

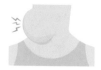

swollen glands

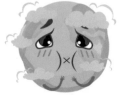

suffocative breathing

hoarseness

anxiety

MENTAL SYMPTOMS
Anxiety
Fear of death from suffocation

EVENT THAT CAUSED SYMPTOMS:
Dry cold weather
Mental excitement

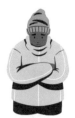

dry cold weather

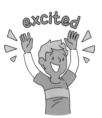

excitement

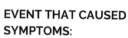

< cold wind

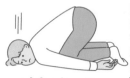

> lying head low

Hindered by:
Dry, cold wind
Warm room
Sweets
Night
Touch
Full moon

Helped by:
Lying with head low
Drinking warm drinks

Spongia
Cheat sheet

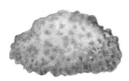

Full name: Spongia Tosta
Other names: Roasted
sponge, Common sponge,
Porifera
Spongia is made from roasted
and triturated sea sponge.

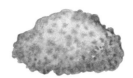

USEFUL FOR:

COUGHS AND RESPIRATORY ISSUES: Dry, barking, croupy cough
resembling the sound of a saw being driven through wood. Cough
worsens at night, with a tickling sensation in the throat. Breathing
difficulties, especially with a feeling of constriction in the chest. Chest
pain with a burning sensation and tightness. Sensation of suffocation or
pressure in the chest. Whooping cough.

CROUP: Use if Aconite fails.

HEART: Palpitations with anxiety and restlessness. Sensation of the
heart pounding in the chest.

THROAT: Enlarged tonsils with a dry, raw, and burning sensation in the
throat. Difficulty swallowing, especially with a sensation of a lump in the
throat. Hoarseness of voice with a dry, raw, and sore throat. Laryngitis
with difficulty speaking.

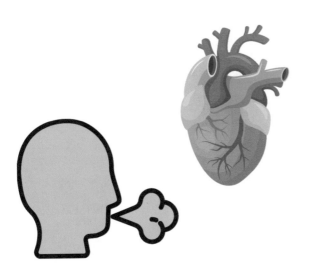

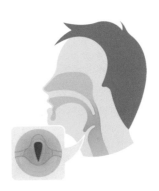

Staphisagria
Suppressed anger, cystitis, styes, lacerated wounds

KEY SYMPTOMS:
- Sensitive to being cut, injured and feeling insulted.
- Styes on the eyelids
- Cystitis especially after sex
- Irritable bladder from suppressed anger
- Crumbling teeth in children
- Hair loss after grief
- Headaches from indignation
- Trembling from anger
- Sleepy all day but sleepless at night
- Abdominal pain after surgery
- Physical cuts and lacerations
- Episiotomy after labour

styes on eyelid

cystitis

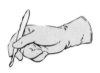

cuts & lacerations

episiotomy after labour

suppressed anger

MENTAL SYMPTOMS
Suppressed emotions and anger
Sweet, suppressed people who draw out sympathy

EVENT THAT CAUSED SYMPTOMS:
Shame
Violation
Punishment
Suppressed anger
Humiliation
Surgery
Lacerations

shame

surgery

< afternoon nap

> warmth

Hindered by:
Touch
Cold drinks
Tobacco
Afternoon naps

Helped by:
Warmth
Rest
Breakfast

Staphisagria
Cheat sheet

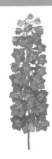

HELP!

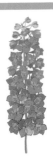

Other names: Stavesacre
Delphinium staphysagria
Made from the seeds of the plant,
Stavesacre. Staphysagria is a perennial
flowering plant which is native to the
Mediterranean region and certain parts
of Asia.

USES FOR:

BLADDER: Cystitis with frequent urging for urine. Burning that is relieved by passing urine. Difficulty passing urine. Pent up anger. Irritable bladder and urging. Cystitis after first sexual intercourse.

FACIAL NEURALGIA: after dentistry

HEADACHES: from suppressed anger. Feels like 'a block of wood' in the forehead.

HEAD LICE: for recurrent infestations that keep coming back despite conventional treatment.

POST SURGERY: For skin wounds and surgical incisions.

STOMACH: Severe pain following operations. Spasmodic cutting pain after eating or drinking. Swollen tummy in children with much wind. Colic after anger.

STYES: Styes on the eyelid. Recurrent styes. Stye doesn't suppurate but remains a hard nodule.

TEETH: Teeth black and crumbling. Teeth decay as soon as they erupt. Toothache. Violent pains into roots. Decay of teeth during pregnancy. Receding gums. Teething in children who are sensitive to mental or physical impressions.

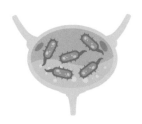

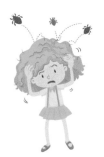

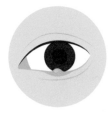

Stramonium
Night terrors, delirious fevers

KEY SYMPTOMS:
- Eyes staring wide open
- Desires light
- Expression of terror
- Aversion to fluids
- Headaches from the sun
- Chorea and spasms
- Stammering
- 'Never been well since' Scarlet Fever
- Night terrors
- Vomiting of green bile
- Violent fevers
- Great thirst yet dreads water

night terrors

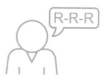

stammering

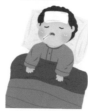

violent fevers

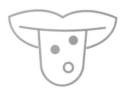

ailments after Scarlet Fever

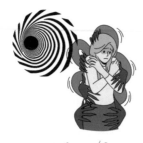

extreme fear

MENTAL SYMPTOMS
Delirium with desire to escape
Mania
Must have light and company
Extreme fear, especially of tunnels

EVENT THAT CAUSED SYMPTOMS:
Shock
Fright
Childbirth
Dog bites
High fever
Head injury

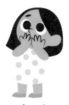

shock

dog bite

< shining object

> bright light

Hindered by:
Shining objects such as water or mirror
Sun
When alone

Helped by:
Bright light
Company

Stramonium
Cheat sheet

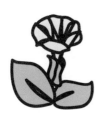

Other names: Jimson Weed, Thornaple, Datura stramonium
Made from the plant Datura stramonium, a tall, annual herbaceous plant that belongs to the Solanaceae family. It is native to North America but has spread to various regions around the world. The plant has large, trumpet-shaped white or purple flowers and spiky fruits containing many seeds.

USEFUL FOR:

ANXIETY: Intense and irrational fears, especially of darkness, death or being alone. Night terrors and nightmares, with a sense of impending doom. Wild and uncontrollable behaviour.

CONVULSIONS: Seizures with violent, jerking movements of the body. Convulsions triggered by fear or emotional excitement. Stammering.

FEVERS: High fevers with extreme restlessness and delirium. Fevers with hallucinations and fear of imaginary objects or creatures.

SLEEP: Number 1 remedy for night terrors. Weeping in dreams. Screaming in sleep. Clings to those near. Must sleep with light on.

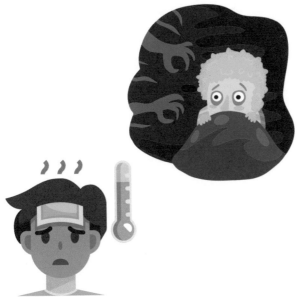

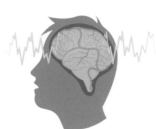

Streptococcinum
Sore throats, strep infections

KEY SYMPTOMS:

- History of strep infections
- Repeated tonsillitis, quinsy or ear infections
- Susceptibility to colds and sore throats
- 'Never been well since' a strep infection
- Arthritis and joint pains
- Sinusitis
- Severe flu, pneumonia, bronchitis or pleurisy
- Homesickness
- Oversensitive
- Sensitive to light and noise

tonsillitis

sinusitis

homesickness

ailments after Strep

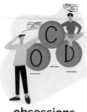

obsessions

MENTAL SYMPTOMS
Depressed
Weeps on being given sympathy
Obsessions
Highly strung

EVENT THAT CAUSED SYMPTOMS:
Strep infections
Tonsillectomy

strep infections

tonsillectomy

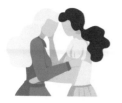

< consolation

> open air

Hindered by:
Consolation
Humid weather
Drafts
Wet weather
First movement

Helped by:
Continued movement
Open air

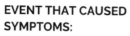

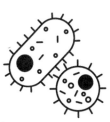 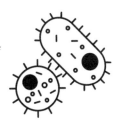

Streptococcinum
Cheat sheet

HELP!

Other names: Streptococcus Nosode, Streptococcinum bacteria
Streptococcinum is a homeopathic remedy made from the bacteria Streptococcus pyogenes. Homeopathic remedies made out of bacteria, and other diseases, are called 'nosodes.'

USEFUL FOR:
GLANDS: Swollen lymph nodes, especially in the neck and throat area. Glandular infections and inflammations.

THROAT: Frequent throat infections. Susceptibility to streptococcal infections, including strep throat. When other well indicated remedies fail to act.

SKIN: Skin problems that worsen or recur after an infection. Eruptions or rashes with a tendency to be sore or inflamed. Cellulitis.

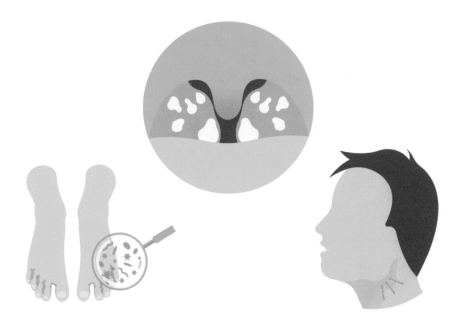

Sulphur
The King of Remedies, skin, relapsing complaints

KEY SYMPTOMS:
- Complaints that relapse
- Warm and aggravated by heat
- Offensive discharges and stools
- Craves sweets and beers
- Empty hungry feeling at 11am
- Dry, burning, hot and itchy skin
- Thirsty for cold drinks
- Diarrhoea every morning driving them out of bed at 5-6am
- Oozing, burning or itching of orifices especially lips and anus

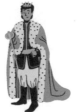

the King of Remedies

complaints that relapse

dry hot itching skin

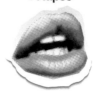

burning orifices esp lips & anus

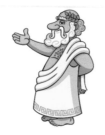

the Ragged Philosopher

MENTAL SYMPTOMS
Dirty or messy - averse to bathing
Absent minded
Bored easily
'Ragged philosopher'
Persistent thoughts

EVENT THAT CAUSED SYMPTOMS:
Suppressions
Alcohol
Sun
Overexertion

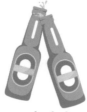

alcohol

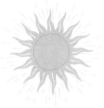

sun

< 11am

> sweating

Hindered by:
11am
Washing
Full moon
Periodically
Suppressions
Milk
Warmth

Helped by:
Dry warm weather
Open air
Sweating
Standing in the most uncomfortable position

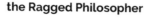

Sulphur
Cheat sheet

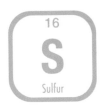

16

S

Sulfur

Other names: Brimstone
Made from the element sulphur.
Sulphur is a naturally occurring non-metallic
element. It is abundant in nature and is found
in various forms. Sulphur is often found in
association with volcanic activity. It can be
found in the form of elemental sulphur near
active or dormant volcanoes, where volcanic
gases containing sulphur compounds are
released.

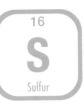

16

S

Sulfur

USEFUL FOR:

COUGHS AND RESPIRATORY ISSUES: Oppression as if a load on the chest.
Chronic cough with thick, yellowish or greenish mucus. Wheezing and
difficulty breathing, especially at night.

FEMALE: Vagina and vulva burn. Menstrual irregularities, such as late or
scanty periods. Hot flashes with hot head, hands and feet. Night sweats
during menopause.

HEMORRHOIDS: Hemorrhoids with burning, itching and stitching pains.
Swollen red anus.

SKIN: Itchy, burning and red skin conditions. Dry, rough, and scaly skin with
a tendency to worsen in heat and bathing. Unhealthy looking skin with
acne or pustules. Burning red orifices.

STOMACH: Gastric disturbances with a sensation of fullness and bloating
after eating. Acid reflux and heartburn, especially after spicy or fatty foods.
Diarrhoea in the morning or after eating. Worms.

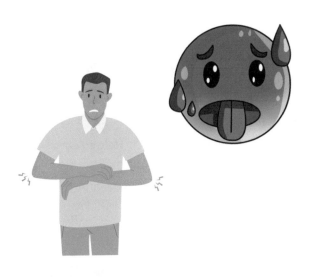

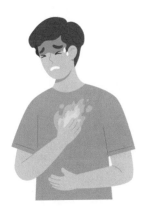

Thuja
Warts, verrucas, sinusitis

KEY SYMPTOMS:

- Medical interventions clouding the picture
- Warts and verrucas
- Herpes
- Fungal growths
- Styes
- Left sided complaints
- Sensation as if something is alive in abdomen or is pregnant
- Headaches like a 'nail driven inward'
- Acne
- Teeth decay at gum line
- Thin eyebrows especially on lateral half
- Chronic sinus issues
- Overproduction of thick yellow/green discharge
- Asthmatic - loose, wet, often 3am/3pm

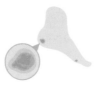

verrucas

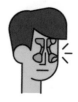

sinusitis

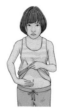

sensation as if something alive in the stomach

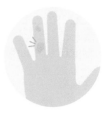

warts

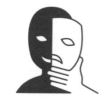

hides behind a mask

MENTAL SYMPTOMS
Secretive - hides behind a mask
Desperate to fit in
Feels they are ugly
Depression and feels alone
Fear of germs

EVENT THAT CAUSED SYMPTOMS:
Tea, coffee, fats, tobacco
Walking
Sexual excess

tea

walking

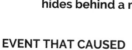

< cold, damp weather

> crossing limbs

Hindered by:
Cold and damp
Night
Moonlight
After urinating

Helped by:
Drawing up limbs
Crossing limbs
Motion
Pressure
Free secretions

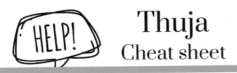

Thuja
Cheat sheet

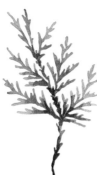

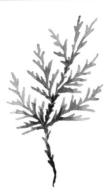

Full name: Thuja Occidentalis
Other names: Arborvitae, White Cedar
Made from the fresh green twigs and leaves of
the tree Thuja occidentalis, commonly known
as Arborvitae or White Cedar. Thuja occidentalis
is an evergreen tree native to North America
and is widely distributed across various regions.
It has scale-like leaves and small cones.

USEFUL FOR:

EYES: Conjunctivitis. Blood red eyes. Full of tears. Styes. Burning and stinging
of eyelids.

FEMALE: Genital warts. Vaginitis. Thick green discharge. Ovarian cysts.
Uterine polyps.

HEADACHES: Headaches with a sensation of a nail or plug in the head.

SKIN: Warts, verrucas, polyps, fungus growths. Warts, especially large,
seedy, or cauliflower-like warts on the face, hands, and genitals. Skin
conditions with a tendency to develop thickened or discoloured patches.
Eruptions with a strong offensive odour.

SINUSITIS: Chronic sinus infections. Catarrh, thick, green-yellow mucus. Nose
is red and hot. Coryza copious outside and dry indoors.

STOMACH: Digestive disturbances with a sensation of a lump or stone in the
stomach. Diarrhoea alternating with constipation.

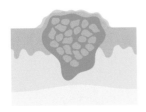

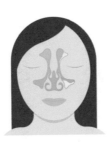

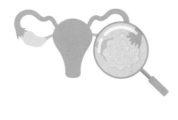

Tuberculinum
Respiratory issues, coughs, tonsillitis

KEY SYMPTOMS:

- Respiratory issues including pneumonia
- Hard, short, dry, constant cough
- Frequent colds and flu
- Reactive asthma (rather than mucus)
- Tonsillitis and enlarged tonsils
- Bedwetting
- Allergies to animal hair and milk
- Glandular problems
- Ringworm
- Consumption (yet looks healthy - red cheeks)
- Headbanging
- Teeth grinding
- Crave smoked meats

respiratory issues

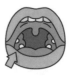

enlarged tonsils

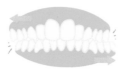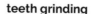

teeth grinding

craves smoked meats

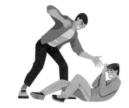

irritable and even violent

MENTAL SYMPTOMS
Easily bored
Hyperactive
Irritable and even violent

EVENT THAT CAUSED SYMPTOMS:
History of tuberculosis in ancestry

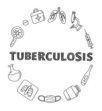

TUBERCULOSIS

< cold, damp weather   > mountain air

Hindered by:
Change of weather
Cold, damp
On waking

Helped by:
Air in the mountains
Pine forests
Warm weather

Tuberculinum
Cheat sheet

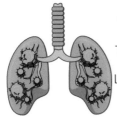
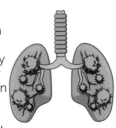

Other names: Tuberculosis Nosode, Tuberculinum of Koch, Tuberculinum bovinum

Tuberculinum is a homeopathic remedy made from the tuberculous sputum or lung tissue of individuals who have been diagnosed with tuberculosis. Homeopathic remedies made out of bacteria, and other diseases, are called 'nosodes.'

USESFUL FOR:

COUGHS AND RESPIRATORY ISSUES: Recurrent respiratory infections, especially involving the lungs. Shortness of breath and difficulty breathing. Chronic cough with greenish or yellowish expectoration. Symptoms which change. Takes cold easily.

GLANDS: Swollen lymph nodes, especially in the neck and under the arms. Glandular infections and inflammations.

THROAT: Hoarseness which is helped by talking. Enlarged tonsils. Hawks mucus after eating. Recurrent tonsillitis.

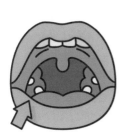
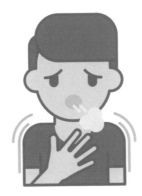
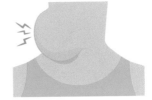

Essential combination remedies

ABC
Injury mix (ARR)
Lisa's 2nd stage mix (MHS)
Post Surgery / Healing mix
Narayani Calming pills
Narayani Coughs, Chest, Asthma (CCA)
Narayani Drawing mix
Narayani War mix

ABC remedy
Fevers, teething, first stage inflammation

USES:

- Any sudden onset first stage inflammations such as sore throats, ear infections, coughs, teething and pain.

CONTAINS (in a 30c):

- ACONITE - for sudden onset inflammations, anxiety, high fevers, pain
- BELLADONNA - for sudden onset inflammation, red, throbbing pain
- CHAMOMILLA - for irritability, anger and extreme sensitivity to pain

DOSING:

- Remember to ALWAYS LISTEN TO THE BODY
- Give every 15-60 minutes and reduce as the symptoms improve
- STOP when definite improvement is maintained
- If you have given 3-4 doses and there is NO improvement then try a different remedy
- If symptoms do return, resume giving the remedy

I CAN'T FIND ABC TO BUY. HOW DO I MAKE IT?!

How to make your own ABC:
Get 1 pill of Aconite 30c, 1 pill of Belladonna 30c and 1 pill of Chamomilla 30c from your standard homeopathy kit and place in a bottle of fresh water. Shake the bottle to dissolve the remedies - do not worry if they do not fully dissolve. One drop or sip of water is equivalent to one pill of pre-mixed ABC. Each time you need to repeat a dose just take another sip of water.

The remedy should stay active in the bottle of water for at least 24 hours.

Injury /ARR mix
For all injuries, sprains and strains

USES:
- For all injuries, sprains and strains. Speeds up healing and prevents bruising.

CONTAINS (in a 30c):
- ARNICA - the universal healing and trauma remedy to speed up healing, reduces inflammation
- RHUS TOX - for sprains and strains and stiffness to joints and muscles. Helped by continued motion and hindered by first movement
- RUTA- used for conditions that involve injuries to tendons, ligaments, and cartilage, such as sprains, strains, and carpal tunnel syndrome. It is also used for eye strain and stiffness in the neck and back. Slightly more deeper acting Rhus Tox

DOSING:
- Remember to ALWAYS LISTEN TO THE BODY
- Give up to three times a day while symptoms are present

I CAN'T FIND INJURY / ARR MIX TO BUY. HOW DO I MAKE IT?!

How to make your own Injury mix:
Get 1 pill of Arnica 30c, 1 pill of Rhus Tox 30c and 1 pill of Ruta 30c from your standard homeopathy kit and place in a bottle of fresh water. Shake the bottle to dissolve the remedies - do not worry if they do not fully dissolve. One drop or sip of water is equivalent to one pill of pre-mixed Injury mix.
Each time you need to repeat a dose just take another sip of water.

The remedy should stay active in the bottle of water for at least 24 hours.

Lisa's 2nd stage mix -MHS
Second stage inflammation, deeper infections

USES:

- Second stage inflammations such as sore throats, ear infections, coughs, teething and pain which have been slower to set in, slow to resolve or with deeper, thicker mucus.

CONTAINS:

- MERC - for infections with foul discharges
- HEPAR SULPH - speeds up suppuration. For thick catarrh
- SILICA - Pulls out morbid material

DOSING:

- Remember to ALWAYS LISTEN TO THE BODY
- Give every 15-60 minutes and reduce as the symptoms improve
- STOP when definite improvement is maintained
- If you have given 3-4 doses and there is NO improvement then try a different remedy
- If symptoms do return, resume giving the remedy

HOW DO I MAKE MY OWN MHS?

How to make your own MHS:
Get 1 pill of Merc 30c, 1 pill of Hepar Sulph 30c
and 1 pill of Silica 30c from your standard homeopathy kit
and place in a bottle of fresh water. Shake the bottle to dissolve the
remedies - do not worry if they do not fully dissolve.
One drop or sip of water is equivalent to one dose.
Each time you need to repeat a dose just take another sip of water.

The remedy should stay active in the bottle of water for at least 24
hours.

Post surgery & healing mix
Use post surgery and post childbirth

USES:
- Speeds up healing (emotionally and physically) and prevents bruising.

CONTAINS (in a 30c or 200c):
- ARNICA - the universal healing and trauma remedy to speed up healing, reduces inflammation
- BELLIS PERENNIS - injuries to deep tissues. Like a deeper acting Arnica.
- CALENDULA - for open wounds, pains. prevents infections and speeds up healing. 'The homeopathic antiseptic'
- HYPERICUM - number 1 post surgery along with Arnica. For damage to nerve rich areas. Known as 'Arnica of the nerves'
- STAPHISAGRIA - for physical violation (including emotional impact) and cutting by sharp instruments

DOSING:
- Remember to ALWAYS LISTEN TO THE BODY
- Give up to three times a day while symptoms are present

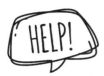

I CAN'T FIND POST SURGERY MIX TO BUY. HOW DO I MAKE IT?!

How to make your own post surgery mix:
Get 1 pill of Arnica 30c, 1 pill of Bellis Perennis 30c, 1 pill of Calendula, 1 pill of Hypericum and 1 pill of Staphisagria from your standard homeopathy kit and place in a bottle of fresh water. Shake the bottle to dissolve the remedies - do not worry if they do not fully dissolve. One drop or sip of water is equivalent to one pill of pre-mixed post surgery mix. Each time you need to repeat a dose just take another sip of water.

The remedy should stay active in the bottle of water for at least 24 hours.

Narayani Calming Pills
Calms the entire system

The Narayani remedies are a powerful set of combination remedies that were put together by a 'classical homeopath'

USES:

- Calms the entire system, both mentally and physically. Also useful for insomnia. After taking the first few doses may want to sleep.

CONTAINS (in a 30c potency):

- AVENA SATIVA - for nervous exhaustion and insomnia
- COFFEA - for insomnia, nervous agitation and restlessness
- HUMULUS - helps dizziness, twitching, nervous tremors and overexcitement
- IGNATIA - for hysteria, grief, depression, sighing, twitching and effects of grief
- KALI PHOS - a nerve tonic for nervous exhaustion, burn out and irritability
- PASSIFLORA - for insomnia, anxiety and stress. It calms and quieten the mind
- SUMBUL - for hysteria, nervousness and palpitations
- VALERIANA - for oversensitivity, hysteria, irritability

DOSING:

- Remember to ALWAYS LISTEN TO THE BODY
- Use when acute symptoms are present
- Give up to three times a day
- In cases of extreme nervousness may increase to six times per day
- For long standing and chronic emotional issues always work with a homeopath

WHERE CAN I BUY NARAYANI MIXES FROM?

Due to the number of non-standard remedies contained within Narayani mixes they should be bought premixed.

See Lisa's website **www.lisastrbac.com** for the most up to date information on remedy stockists.

Narayani CCA Mix
Coughs, Chest & Asthma (CCA)

The Narayani remedies are a powerful set of combination remedies that were put together by a 'classical homeopath'

USES:

- For all coughs, chest issues and asthma symptoms. Useful when it is not possible to choose an individual remedy.

CONTAINS (in a 30c potency):

- ANT TART - for rattling chest with mucus which is difficult to bring up
- BRONCHI - organ support remedy for bronchi
- BRYONIA - for dry hacking coughs, stitching pain in chest and difficult breathing
- IPECAC - for wheezing and rattling chest. For croup and whooping cough
- KALI BICH - for yellow, sticky and stringy discharges. For croup and hacking coughs
- MUCUS MEMBRANES - organ support remedy for mucus membranes
- NAT SULPH - great chest remedy, thick and yellow expectorant
- RUMEX - for dry coughs which stops sleep
- SULPHUR - for burning in chest, rattling mucus and difficult breathing

DOSING:

- Remember to ALWAYS LISTEN TO THE BODY
- When acute symptoms are present may use up to six times per day
- When symptoms ease, reduce to up to three times a day for up to seven days

WHERE CAN I BUY NARAYANI MIXES FROM?

Due to the number of non-standard remedies contained within Narayani mixes they should be bought premixed.

See Lisa's website **www.lisastrbac.com** for the most up to date information on remedy stockists.

Narayani Drawing Mix
Helps to draw out infections

USES:

- Draws out infections. Mucus anywhere in the body is pulled out - sinus, tonsils, ears, uterus or rectum. Boils and carbuncles matured. Fissures and ulcers drained. Works even for longstanding issues.

CONTAINS (in a 6x potency):

- HEPAR SULPH - speeds up suppuration
- GUNPOWDER - holds infection and prevents it from going deeper
- MYRISTICA SEB - antiseptic action which quickens suppuration and duration
- SILICA - pulls out morbid material

DOSING:

- Remember to ALWAYS LISTEN TO THE BODY
- When acute infections are present use up to six times per day. Reduce to three times a day when suppuration begins
- Can be used alongside any other remedies. As this is in a low potency (6x), it works more on a material level, similar to a supplement or cell/tissue salt, and as such can be dosed more frequently

WHERE CAN I BUY NARAYANI MIXES FROM?

Due to the number of non-standard remedies contained within Narayani mixes they should be bought premixed.

See Lisa's website **www.lisastrbac.com** for the most up to date information on remedy stockists.

Narayani War Mix
Intense infections & inflammation

USES:

- Use for infections and inflammations anywhere in the body.

CONTAINS (in a 1m potency):

- PENICILLIN - reported by Narayani to work in the same way as the allopathic antibiotic but without any side effects
- BELLADONNA - for red, throbbing inflammations
- GUNPOWDER - holds infection and prevents it from going deeper
- CORTISONE - reported by Narayani to work in the same way as the allopathic version but without any side effects. Helps with pain
- STREPTOCOCCUS - a homeopathic remedy made from streptococcus.
- STAPHYLOCOCCUS - a homeopathic remedy made from staphlococcus
- PYROGENIUM - for septic states, pain, burning in wounds or organs, septicaemia or any inflammation
- KALI PHOS - for decay and gangrene

DOSING:

- Remember to ALWAYS LISTEN TO THE BODY
- When acute infections are present can use up to six times per day for the first day, then may take up to three times a day for up to five days

WHERE CAN I BUY NARAYANI MIXES FROM?

Due to the number of non-standard remedies contained within Narayani mixes they should be bought premixed.

See Lisa's website **www.lisastrbac.com** for the most up to date information on remedy stockists.

Index of symptoms

Index of symptoms

Accidents & injuries
Injury mix
Aconite
Arnica
Bellis Perennis
Calendula
Hypericum
Ledum
Rhus Tox
Ruta

Allergies/ Hives/Itching
Allium cepa
Apis
Dolichos
Euphrasia
Histaminum
Rhus Tox
Sulphur

Anxiety
Narayani Calming
Aconite
Ambra grisea
Anacardium
Arg Nit
Arsenicum
Calc carb
Gelsemium
Kali Phos
Lycopodium
Phosphorus
Stramonium

Bites, stings & splinters
Narayani Drawing
Apis
Belladonna
Cantharis
Histaminum
Hypericum
Lachesis
Ledum
Silica

Bladder infection
Narayani Drawing
Narayani War
Apis
Cantharis
Causticum
Merc
Nat Mur
Nux Vom
Pulsatilla
Staphisagria

Boils & abscesses
Narayani Drawing
Narayani War
MHS mix
Belladonna
Bellis Perennis
Hepar Sulph
Lachesis
Merc
Silica
Sulphur

Burns
Surgery/Healing mix
Apis
Arsenicum
Belladonna
Calendula
Cantharis
Causticum
Hypericum
Rhus Tox

Chicken pox
Aconite
Ant Tart
Apis
Belladonna
Histaminum
Merc
Pulsatilla
Rhus Tox
Sulphur

Index of symptoms

Childbirth
Surgery/Healing mix
Aconite
Arnica
Belladonna
Bellis Perennis
Calendula
Caulophyllum
Chamomilla
Cimicifuga
Gelsemium
Kali Carb
Secale

Cold sores
MHS mix
Narayani Drawing
Arsenicum
Hepar Sulph
Merc
Nat Mur
Rhus Tox
Sepia

Colds
ABC
Narayani Drawing
Aconite
Allium cepa
Arsenicum
Calc Carb
Euphrasia
Ferrum Phos
Kali Bich
Nat Mur
Nux Vom
Pulsatilla

Colic
ABC
Arg Nit
Belladonna
Bryonia
Calc Phos
Carbo Veg
Chamomilla
Colocynthis
Lycopodium
Nux Vom
Staphisagria

Collapse
Arnica
China
Carbo Veg

Conjunctivitis
Narayani Drawing
Narayani War
Apis
Arg Nit
Belladonna
Euphrasia
Merc
Pulsatilla
Rhus Tox
Thuja

Constipation
Aesculus
Bryonia
Calc Carb
Dolichos
Lycopodium
Nat Mur
Nux Vom
Opium
Sepia
Silica

Index of symptoms

Coughs
Narayani CCA
Aconite
Ambra grisea
Ant Tart
Arsenicum
Bryonia
Causticum
Drosera
Eupatorium
Ferrum Phos
Hepar Sulph
Ignatia
Ipecac
Kali Bich
Kali Carb
Phosphorus
Pulsatilla
Spongia
Sulphur
Tuberculinum

Cramps
Belladonna
Calc Phos
Chamomilla
Colocynthis
Mag Phos
Nux Vom

Croup
Narayani CCA
Aconite
Drosera
Hepar Sulph
Kali Bich
Phosphorus
Spongia

Diarrhoea
Arg Nit
Arsenicum
Carbo Veg
Chamomilla
China
Gelsemium
Nux Vom
Phos Ac
Phosphorus
Sulphur

Ear infection
ABC
MHS mix
Narayani Drawing
Narayani War
Aconite
Belladonna
Calc Carb
Capsicum
Chamomilla
Ferrum Phos
Hepar Sulph
Merc
Pulsatilla
Silica

Exhaustion
Narayani Calming
Ambra grisea
Anacardium
Arsenicum
Carbo veg
China
Gelsemium
Kali Phos
Phos Ac
Phosphorus
Sepia

Index of symptoms

Fevers
ABC
Narayani Drawing
Narayani War
Aconite
Arsenicum
Belladonna
Bryonia
Chamomilla
Ferrum Phos
Gelsemium
Phosphorus
Pulsatilla
Stramonium

Flu
Narayani CCA
Narayani Drawing
Narayani War
Aconite
Ant Tart
Arsenicum
Belladonna
Bryonia
Eupatorium
Ferrum Phos
Gelsemium
Ipecac
Nux Vom
Rhus Tox

Gout
Ledum

Grief
Narayani Calming
Causticum
Ignatia
Nat Mur
Phos Ac
Pulsatilla

Growing pains
Calc Phos
Mag Phos

Hand, foot and mouth
Arsenicum
Merc
Rhus Tox

Hayfever
Allium cepa
Arsenicum
Euphrasia
Histaminum
Mixed pollens
Nat Mur
Nux Vom
Pulsatilla
Sabadilla

Headaches
Ambra grisea
Anacardium
Arg Nit
Belladonna
Bryonia
Eupatorium
Ferrum Phos
Gelsemium
Ignatia
Kali Bich
Kali Phos
Lachesis
Nat Mur
Nux Vom
Phosphorus
Pulsatilla
Silica
Staphisagria
Thuja

Index of symptoms

Hemorrhoids
Aesculus
Capsicum
Dolichos
Nux Vom
Sulphur

Impetigo
Narayani War
Arsenicum
Merc
Rhus Tox
Silica

Indigestion
Arg Nit
Arsenicum
Bryonia
Carbo veg
China
Lycopodium
Nux Vom
Pulsatilla
Staphisagria
Sulphur

Insomnia
Narayani Calming
Ambra grisea
Arsenicum
Calc Carb
Chamomilla
Cocculus
Kali Phos
Nux Vom
Opium
Phos Ac

Jet lag
Arnica
Cocculus

Joint pains
Injury mix
Aesculus
Arnica
Bellis Perennis
Caulophyllum
Causticum
Kali Bich
Phytolacca
Rhus Tox
Ruta

Liver
Aesculus
Chelidonium
Dolichos
Lycopodium
Nux Vom

Mastitis
Narayani Drawing
Narayani War
Belladonna
Bryonia
Hepar Sulph
Merc
Phytolacca

Measles
Aconite
Apis
Belladonna
Bryonia
Euphrasia
Gelsemium
Pulsatilla
Sulphur

Menopause
Belladonna
Cimicifuga
Lachesis
Pulsatilla
Sepia
Sulphur

Index of symptoms

Molluscum Contagiosum
Silica
Thuja

Morning sickness
Arsenicum
Cocculus
Ipecac
Nux Vom
Pulsatilla
Sepia

Mumps
Aconite
Apis
Belladonna
Calc Carb
Lachesis
Phytolacca
Pulsatilla

Nausea & vomiting
Ant Tart
Arsenicum
Bryonia
Carbo veg
China
Cocculus
Ipecac
Nux Vom
Phosphorus
Pulsatilla
Sepia

Nightmares
Calc Carb
Cina
Phosphorus
Stramonium

Nosebleeds
Arnica
Ferrum Phos
Phosphorus

Period pains
Narayani Calming
Belladonna
Chamomilla
Cimiciguga
Cocculus
Colocynthis
Lachesis
Lycopodium
Mag phos
Nat Mur
Nux Vom
Pulsatilla
Secale
Sepia

Respiratory
Narayani CCA
Ant Tart
Arsenicum
Carbo veg
Causticum
China
Drosera
Eupatorium
Ferrum Phos
Hepar Sulph
Ipecac
Kali Bich
Kali Carb
Lachesis
Phosphorus
Pulsatilla
Spongia
Sulphur
Tuberculinum

Rubella (German measles)
Aconite
Pulsatilla

Index of symptoms

Sciatica
Injury mix
Aesculus
Arnica
Arsenicum
Bryonia
Colocynthis
Gelsemium
Hypericum
Kali Carb
Lycopodium
Mag phos
Phytolacca
Rhus Tox
Ruta

Sepsis
Narayani Drawing
Narayani War

Shingles
Apis
Arsenicum
Rhus Tox

Shock
Narayani Calming
Aconite
Arnica
Gelsemium
Ignatia
Opium

Sinusitis
MHS mix
Narayani Drawing
Narayani War
Bryonia
Hepar Sulph
Kali Bich
Merc
Pulsatilla
Silica
Thuja

Sprains & strains
Injury mix
Arnica
Bellis Perennis
Bryonia
Hypericum
Ledum
Rhus tox
Ruta

Styes
MHS mix
Narayani Drawing
Narayani War
Apis
Hepar Sulph
Pulsatilla
Silica
Staphisagria
Thuja

Sunburn
Apis
Belladonna
Calendula
Cantharis

Surgery
Surgery/Healing mix
Arnica
Bellis Perennis
Calendula
Hypericum
Phosphorus
Staphisagria

Index of symptoms

Teething
ABC
Aconite
Belladonna
Calc Carb
Calc Phos
Chamomilla
Mag Phos
Pulsatilla

**Throat Issues &
Tonsillitis**
MHS mix
Narayani Drawing
Narayani War
Aconite
Apis
Arg Nit
Belladonna
Cantharis
Capsicum
Causticum
Ferrum Phos
Ignatia
Lachesis
Lycopodium
Merc
Phosphorus
Phytolacca
Silica
Spongia
Streptococcinum
Tuberculinum

Thrush
Arsenicum
Candida Albicans
Capsicum
Merc
Nat Mur

Travel sickness
Arnica
Bryonia
China
Cocculus
Nux Vom
Pulsatilla

Varicose Veins
Aesculus
Bellis Perennis
Carbo veg
Lachesis
Pulsatilla

Vertigo
Bryonia
Cocculus
Gelsemium

Warts
Causticum
Thuja

Whooping cough
Narayani CCA
Ant Tart
Cina
Drosera
Ipecac
Spongia

Worms / Parasites
Cina
Dolichos
Sabadilla
Sulphur

Wounds
Surgery / Healing mix
Arnica
Calendula
Hypericum
Ledum

About Lisa Strbac
LCHE BSc(Hons)

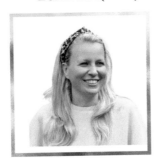

I'm a certified Homeopath LCHE BSc (Hons) and an ambassador for my profession. I'm passionate about empowering the individual to take responsibility for their own health, with the understanding that true health comes from within. Learning how to use homeopathy in the home is one of the most transformational steps an individual can make for their own and their family's health.

My journey towards holistic health started in 2015, after witnessing the power of homeopathy to heal my then 5 year old daughter's chronic autoimmune condition. I was a previous sceptic but I had exhausted all conventional approaches. I was so awestruck with homeopathy that I had to learn more, and, after 4 years of study and clinical practice, I obtained my Licentiate from the UK's largest accredited college, The Centre for Homeopathic Education. I am also an Integrative Nutrition Health Coach, having studied at The Institute of Integrative Nutrition, the world's largest health coaching and nutrition school.

My 'work' has evolved to teaching individuals on how to use homeopathy at home and I run a variety of very popular homeopathy online courses, which my attendees have described as 'life changing.' If every individual had a basic homeopathy kit and knew how to use it, the world would be a very different place.

We could avoid so many health issues if we understood how to naturally support health rather than suppress symptoms - homeopathy is amazing for this and there really is nothing else out there quite like it.

For more information on me and my courses you can connect with me at **www.lisastrbac.com.**

Lisa Strbac